50 Ophthalmic Case Studies

Clinical Features and Management

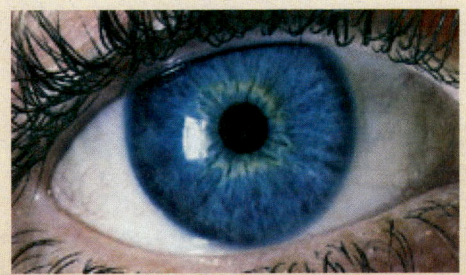

50 Ophthalmic Case Studies

Clinical Features and Management

Sanjeev Agarwal MS

Professor and Head
Department of Ophthalmology
Gandhi Medical College
Bhopal, MP

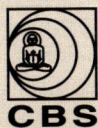

CBS

CBS Publishers & Distributors Pvt Ltd

New Delhi • Bengaluru • Chennai • Kochi • Kolkata • Mumbai
Hyderabad • Jharkhand • Nagpur • Patna • Pune • Uttarakhand

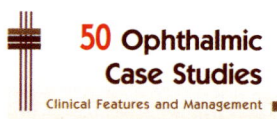

50 Ophthalmic Case Studies

Clinical Features and Management

ISBN: 978-93-86827-91-3

Copyright © Author and Publisher

First Edition: 2018

Published by Satish Kumar Jain and produced by Varun Jain for

CBS Publishers & Distributors Pvt Ltd

4819/XI Prahlad Street, 24 Ansari Road, Daryaganj, New Delhi 110 002, India.
Ph: 23289259, 23266861, 23266867 Website: www.cbspd.com
Fax: 011-23243014 e-mail: delhi@cbspd.com; cbspubs@airtelmail.in.
Corporate Office: 204 FIE, Industrial Area, Patparganj, Delhi 110 092

Ph: 4934 4934 Fax: 4934 4935 e-mail: publishing@cbspd.com; publicity@cbspd.com

Branches

- **Bengaluru:** Seema House 2975, 17th Cross, K.R. Road,
  Banasankari 2nd Stage, Bengaluru 560 070, Karnataka
  Ph: +91-80-26771678/79 Fax: +91-80-26771680 e-mail: bangalore@cbspd.com
- **Chennai:** 7, Subbaraya Street, Shenoy Nagar, Chennai 600 030, Tamil Nadu
  Ph: +91-44-26680620, 26681266 Fax: +91-44-42032115 e-mail: chennai@cbspd.com
- **Kochi:** Ashana House, No. 39/1904, AM Thomas Road, Valanjambalam,
  Ernakulam 682 016, Kochi, Kerala
  Ph: +91-484-4059061-65 Fax: +91-484-4059065 e-mail: kochi@cbspd.com
- **Kolkata:** 6/B, Ground Floor, Rameswar Shaw Road, Kolkata-700 014, West Bengal
  Ph: +91-33-22891126, 22891127, 22891128 e-mail: kolkata@cbspd.com
- **Mumbai:** 83-C, Dr E Moses Road, Worli, Mumbai-400018, Maharashtra
  Ph: +91-22-24902340/41 Fax: +91-22-24902342 e-mail: mumbai@cbspd.com

Representatives

- **Hyderabad** 0-9885175004 • **Jharkhand** 0-9811541605 • **Nagpur** 0-9021734563
- **Patna** 0-9334159340 • **Pune** 0-9623451994 • **Uttarakhand** 0-9716462459

Printed at International Print-O-Pac Limited, Noida, UP, India

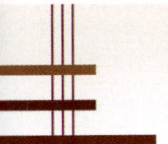

Preface

I have recently updated our old book *Clinical Examinaton of Ophthamic Cases* as third edition mainly aimed at postgraduate students, as coauthor with Prof ML Agarwal. I have also coauthored another book with Prof ML Agarwal *Clinical Presentation of Ophthalmic Cases* mainly for undergraduate students. Both the books cover more than 90% of ophthalmic maladies in a poetic format so that it can be read and digested with ease.

Most of the patients attending outpatient department are easily handled by postgraduate students and faculty as they present with specific symptoms. Among these cases, an ophthalmologist also encounters a few cases who make us scratch our head to conclude diagnosis. These cases need further investigations and indoor admission to conclude the malady and provide treatment.

Keeping this in mind, I am presenting this new book **50 Ophthalmic Case Studies** covering:

- **1–20** Cases with Specific Uncommon Symptomatic Cases
- **21–40** Cases with Specific Common Symptomatic Cases   and
- **41–50** Cases with Common Spot Diagnostic Cases.

These **50 Cases** cover most of the cases encountered by postgraduate students/ residents and the faculty in their day-to-day outpatient clinics in a hospital or a practitioner in private consultation.

This handy book will serve as a "ready-reckoner" in day-to-day life for postgraduate students, faculty and young ophthalmologists in practice.

Sanjeev Agarwal

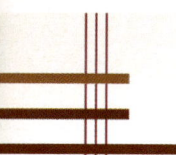

Introduction to Regenerative Ophthalmology with Stem Cell Therapy

Stem cells are the undifferentiated cells which have capacity of self-renewal and differentiation. They are present in all multicellular organisms. Alexander Moximov was the Russian haematologist who postulated about stem cells.

Stem cell treatment is a conceptual change in the treatment of those diseases in which the outcome of disease is poor and cannot be treated by existing modalities of treatment. For most of the ophthalmic maladies like optic atrophy, age-related macular degeneration, retinitis pigmentosa, corneal opacity and corneal degeneration/atrophy in which the patient leads a vegetative life and is considered to be a burden on the family and society, the stem cell therapy or regenerative therapy helps them to regain vision to an extent that they can led life without being burden on the family or the society.

Kindly refer to my chapter in this book titled "Case 20: Regenerative ophthalmology" for more details on stem cell therapy for regeneration of eye tissue.

Mayank Jain
Stem Cell Specialist

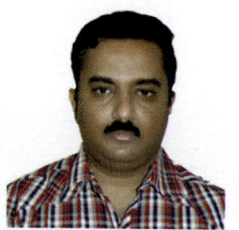

Dr Mayank Jain
(Stem Cell Specialist)

Author Dr Mayank Jain completed post-graduation in 1993. From last 5 years he is into the laboratory research and clinical transfer of stem cells and had done successful clinical transfers in ophthalmic cases also with good results. He had coined a *physiological classification and clinical classification* known as **Mayanks' classification** for stem cells and this classification had become a guideline for stem cell transfer. Author had spearheaded the concept of autologus transfer and condemns allogenic transfer because of ethical issues and its inherent disadvantages. This would bring an end to commercialization of stem cells by various agencies. Presently he is working on role of stem cells in cerebral palsy. Presented paper in international conference on stem cells.

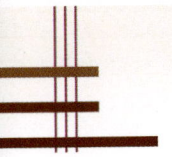

Contents

Part 1
Specific Uncommon Symptomatic Cases

Part 2
Specific Common Symptomatic Cases

Part 3
Common Spot Diagnostic Cases

Part
1

Specific Uncommon
Symptomatic Cases

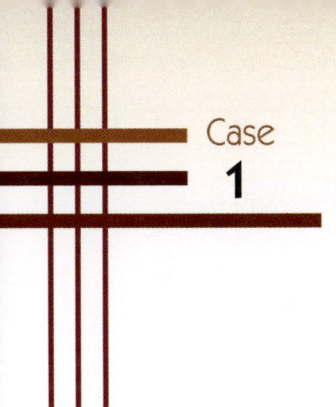

Chiasmal Lesions

Patient enters the clinic with history of headache for a few days. His wife complains that her husband stumbles with the objects in the home and with objects and subjects also while walking.

Confrontation test for field defect reveals bitemporal field defect.

Diagnosis: Chiasmal lesion

CHIASMAL LESIONS

From the ophthalmological point of view early diagnosis and treatment of the chiasmal lesions is of utmost importance as these lesions affect the vision of the patient early with unrecoverability of visual acuity if lost (Fig. 1.1).

The primary main symptom of chiasmal lesion is visual field defect with loss of vision due to optic atrophy (Fig. 1.2).

Typical field defect is bitemporal hemianopia. With a bilateral defect there is no problem in the diagnosis. The problem arises when the defect in unilateral and quadrantic in early stage.

There is gradual visual loss which may not be noticed by the patient. By the time the optic atrophy manifests on ophthalmoscopy it is already too late to recover the lost vision.

Clinical Examination

• *General and systemic examination*: It is a must in every case wherein there is suspicion for chiasmal lesion, especially pituitary lesion. It will help to detect and diagnose any endocrine disorder or syndrome associated with pituitary adenoma.

• *Visual acuity*: It may be normal or low if optic atrophy sets in.

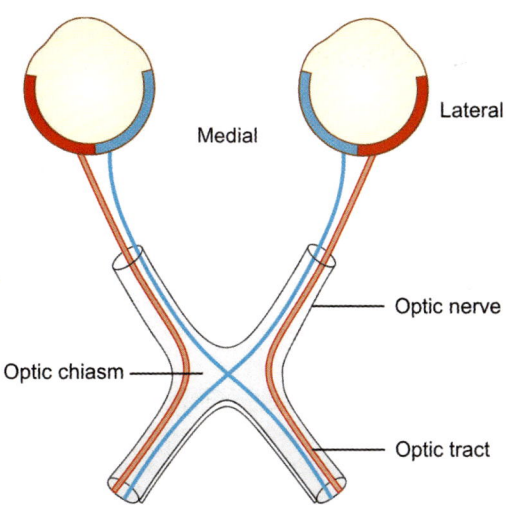

Fig. 1.1: Optic nerve, chiasm and tract

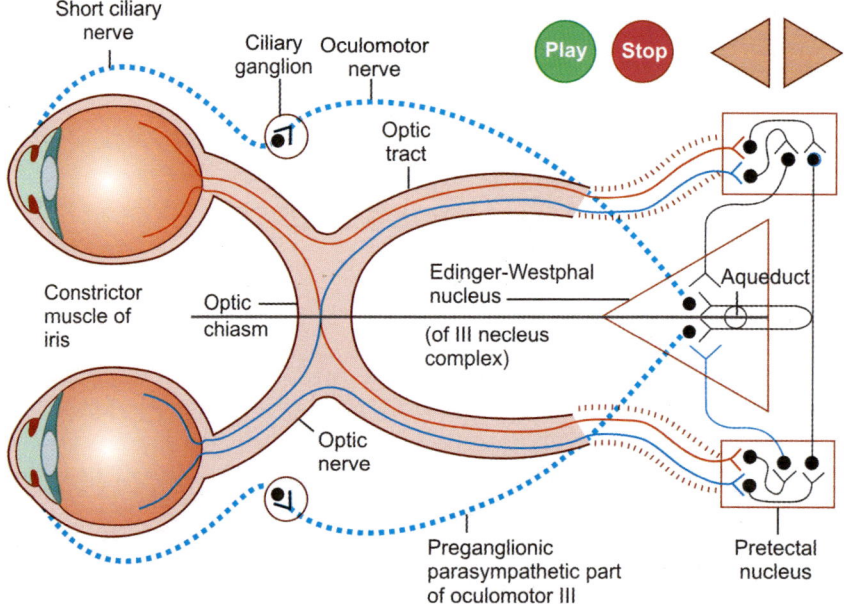

Fig. 1.2: Optic nerve pathway

- *Ophthalmoscopy*: It may show normal fundus or signs of early optic atrophy. Optic atrophy is the most common manifestation of chiasmal lesions.
- *Visual field charting*: Chiasmal lesions always demonstrate visual field defect. Typical bitemporal hemianopia is diagnostic.
- *Ocular movements*: Patients with chiasmal lesions may show ophthalmoplegia of varying degrees.
- *Exophthalmometry*: It is required in cases with proptosis. It is helpful in assessing the prognosis.

Clinical Investigations

Radiography

X-ray skull lateral view for pituitary fossa shall be very helpful (Fig. 1.3). X-ray may be normal. Usually, the sellae is uniformly enlarged with ballooned depression downwards, forwards along with erosion of clinoid process giving the sellae typical *'flattened appearance'*.

i. *In a case of chromophobe adenoma*: The enlargement of sellae is greatest postero-anteriorly with attenuated walls and destroyed clinoid processes first anterior

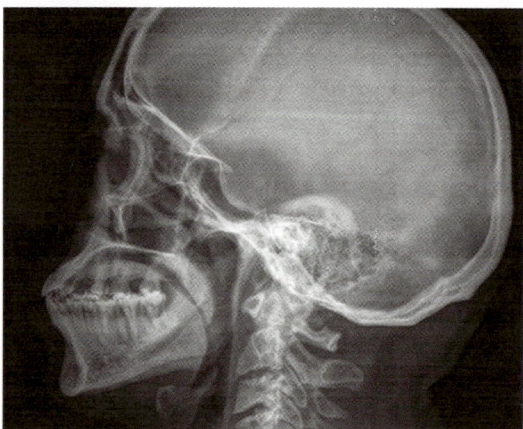

Fig.1.3: Flattened pituitary fossa

and thereafter posterior. It is to be kept in mind that posterior clinoid process may be absent congenitally.

ii. *In acidophil adenoma*: The walls of sellae are thick, sellae and clinoid process not affected and the orifice remains narrower.

Computerized Tomography Scanning

Computerized tomographic scanning is very helpful in exactly localizing the lesion. It shall give very clear outline of sellae with soft tissues also.

Magnetic Resonance Imaging

It is very sensitive for detecting differences between normal and abnormal tissues. It provides better image resolution (Fig. 1.4).

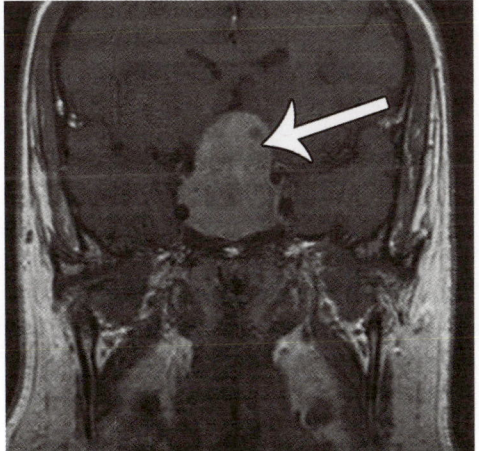

Fig. 1.4: MRI of large pituitary tumor

Ultrasonography

It is helpful in proper assessment of orbital lesion.

CLINICAL FEATURES AND MANAGEMENT

1. *Pituitary adenomas*: Chromophobe, acidophil, mixed and basophil adenoma and Fröhlich's syndrome, gigantism, acromegaly and Cushing's syndrome
2. Pituitary adenocarcinoma
3. Pituitary metastatic tumors
4. Craniopharyngioma (Fröhlich's syndrome, Lorain's type of infantilism, Simmond's pituitary cachexia)
5. Suprasellar meningioma (dural endothelioma)
6. Glioma of chiasma
7. Chiasmal neuritis
8. Chiasmal arachnoiditis
9. Supraclinoid aneurysm (aneurysm of internal carotid artery)
10. Visual field defects associated with chiasmal lesions; (infra-chiasmatic, supra-chiasmatic, peri-chiasmatic and intra-chiasmatic lesions).

1. PITUITARY ADENOMA

Pituitary adenomas are classified as follows:

i. *Chromophobe adenoma*

- It is composed of chromophobe cells of normal gland.
- It is the most common adenoma of pituitary gland manifesting in adults (Fig. 1.5).
- Onset is slow and insidious.
- Only symptom complained by the patient is 'headahce'.
- No other ocular signs or symptoms.
- Radiography shows normal pituitary fossa.
- Chromophobe adenoma is associated with symptoms of hypopituitarism and may present the signs and symptoms of 'Fröhlich's syndrome' (dystrophia adiposogenitalis).

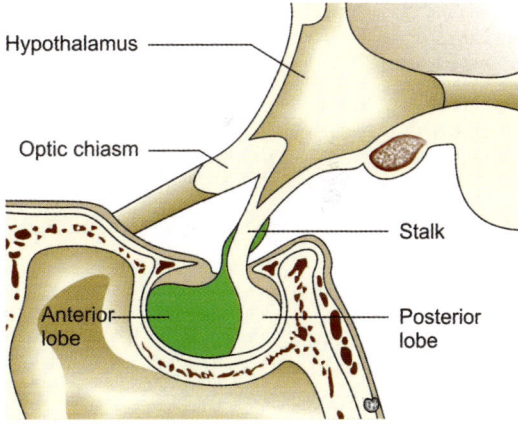

Fig.1.5: Pituitary gland

Clinical features of 'Fröhlich's syndrome'

- Obesity around shoulders and hips
- Soft hairless skin
- Genital hypoplasia
- Impairment of dark adaptation
- Associated symptoms of increased sugar tolerance
- Polyuria, lethargy and narcolepsy are due to damage of tuberal region and second floor of third ventricle along with adenoma.
- Chromophobe adenoma may grow rapidly due to cystic degeneration and

hemorrhage in the tumor then the local signs of tumor will appear.

ii. *Acidophil adenoma*

- It is composed of eosinophil cells of the anterior lobe of pituitary gland.
- It grows very slowly.
- It is associated with symptoms of hyper-pituitarism that manifest as *'gigantism'* in young age and as *'acromegaly'* in the adult.
- It takes years for manifestation of the symptoms of hyperpituitarism. Ocular signs and symptoms arise only when the tumor has become suprasellar affecting the chiasma.

Gigantism

It occurs due to hyperpituitarism in young before their epiphyseal lines are closed. It is characterized by excessive growth at the epiphyseal lines and associated with genital hypoplasia and impotence.

Acromegaly

It also occurs due to hyperpituitarism in adult after the epiphyseal lines are closed.

Clinical features are characteristic over growth of skeletal system such as:

- Enlarged skull and orbits
- Lower jaw becomes prognathous
- Hands and feet are large and spade like
- Hyperosteoses on the terminal phalanges
- Skin is rough with hypertrichosis in both sexes
- Impaired sexual function with impotence in males and amenorrhea in females
- Hyperglycemia and glycosuria
- Increased metabolic rate
- Splanchnomegaly with hypertrophy of many viscera
- Digestive problems

Ocular signs are as follows:

- Defect in visual field
- Optic atrophy
- Proptosis
- Ocular motor palsies.

Clinical picture of acromegaly is so characteristic that after seeing a case, one cannot miss the case thereafter anytime in his life.

iii. *Mixed adenoma*

- Mixed adenoma of pituitary is very rare.
- These are composed of chromophobe and acidophil cells.
- Clinically the symptoms are mixed for hyper- and hypopituitarism.

iv. *Basophil adenoma*

- Basophil adenoma is rarity.
- These occur in young women and are associated with metabolic disorders and fatal within 5 years.
- Along with pituitary dyscrasia there is hyperadrenalism resulting in *'Cushing's syndrome'*.

Clinical features of 'Cushing's syndrome'

- Painful plethoric adiposity
- Cutaneous striae
- Purpuric patches
- Overgrowth of hairs
- Amenorrhea
- Osteoporosis
- Albuminuria.

2. PITUITARY ADENOCARCINOMA

- Adenocarcinoma is a rare tumor of pituitary.
- It is a locally malignant tumor with tendency to destroy the base of skull, bursts through the floor of the sellae and spreads backwards into the third ventricle.
- No metastasis.

3. PITUITARY METASTATIC TUMORS

These are rare. The most common tumor which gets metastatized to pituitary is the carcinoma of breast in the females.

Clinical Features of Pituitary Tumors

1. *Endocrine disorders*

- Fröhlich's syndrome
- Gigantism

- Acromegaly
- Cushing's syndrome

2. *Pressure symptoms of tumor manifests as*

- Headache
- Visual field defects
- Exophthalmos
- Ophthalmoplegia
- Increased intracranial pressure
- Symptoms due to pressure on neighbouring structures.

Headache

It is the first symptom complained by the patient with pituitary tumor. In early stage, headache is due to expansion of sellae. Headache may be severe bursting type either bitemporal or frontal in its distribution.

After destruction of sellae the headache is due to raised intracranial pressure and this time it is associated with vomiting.

Headache may be also due to involvement of fifth nerve.

Visual field defects

Typical field defect is classical 'bitemporal hemianopia'.

The field defect progresses typically—to begin with there is loss of upper quadrant of temporal field on both the sides followed by bitemporal hemianopia. Thereafter gradual loss of the nasal field in the first affected eye resulting in complete blindness in this eye with temporal hemianopia in other eye and finally the nasal field of the other eye is also lost resulting in complete blindness in both the eyes.

As there is a great variation in the relation of the chiasma to the pituitary so many kinds of diversities in the defect of visual field can be expected depending on which part of the chiasma is being pressed by tumor. The presence of field defect indicates that the tumor is pressing upon the chiasma or blood vessels supplying the chiasma.

A slowly progressive tumor will give rise to slow changes in the fields. Pituitary tumor may grow to an enormous size without causing much damage to fields.

Thus field defect only indicates the presence of tumor but neither its size nor its location whether the tumor mass is prefixed or post-fixed, whether the tumor is growing laterally into the middle fossa or growing posteriorly without implicating the chiasma and without field changes or visual impairment.

The only way an ophthalmologist can save vision and further loss of field of vision is to provide relief from pressure by involving *neurosurgeon*. Relief from pressure is likely to improve the vision and fields both if the defect has not lasted long.

'Optic atrophy' is the result of either direct pressure over the optic nerve or it follows papilledema as postpapilledematous optic atrophy.

Only pallor of the optic disc is due to ischemia and has no relation with the visual acuity.

Exophthalmos

It may occur due to disturbance of thyrotropic hormone.

Ophthalmoplegia

Partial ophthalmoplegia may occur due to lateral extension of growth through the walls of cavernous sinus.

Patient may present with simple ptosis or ocular palsies due to involvement of third and fourth cranial nerves.

Ophthalmoplegia may be unilateral or even bilateral.

Total ophthalmoplegia is rarity.

Neuralgia associated with pituitary tumor could be due to involvement of fifth cranial nerve.

Increased intracranial pressure

It occurs after the tumor has destroyed the sellae. It causes headache with vomiting.

Symptoms due to pressure on neighbouring structures

Symptoms may arise by pressure on hypothalamus, temporal and frontal lobe.

Pressure on the hypothalamus can give rise to symptoms such as disturbance in fluid, fat and sugar metabolism, irregular pyrexia, and narcolepsy.

Pressure on the uncinate gyrus of temporal lobe produces uncinate fits with characteristic aura of taste and smell.

Pressure on the frontal lobe causes mental deterioration with abnormal emotional reactions.

Differential Diagnosis

1. Meningioma of lesser wing of sphenoid
2. Aneurysm
3. Tumor of posterior fossa
4. Chiasmal arachnoiditis
5. Optic neuritis.

Management

It is surgical.
Involve neuro-surgeon.

4. CRANIOPHARYNGIOMA

Craniopharyngioma is supra-sellar congenital tumor/cyst that arises from remnants of the epithelial tract from which Rathke's pharyngeal pouch, the anterior lobe of the pituitary and hypophyseal duct are formed.

The growth is usually an epidermoid carcinoma.

Formation of cyst is common.

The tumor may vary from small cysts of peanut size to large calcified multi-cystic mass of the size of tennis ball.

As a rule symptoms appear in childhood or adolescence.

Frequently, it may remain small and stationary for years until adult life.

Characteristic symptoms of chiasmal syndrome— characterized by:

- Optic atrophy
- Bitemporal hemianopia
- No evidence of distention of sella turcica
- Symptoms due to pressure on neighbouring structures with endocrine disturbances of varied type.

Clinical Features and Management

Loss of vision due to optic atrophy

The visual loss is gradual often over period of years.

The optic disc appears normal or pale and the clear picture of optic atrophy manifests late.

Some cases may show papilledema due to encroachment of tumor on the third ventricle causing raised intracranial pressure. Such patient may complain of diplopia due to involvement of the third or sixth cranial nerves.

Usually, both the eyes are affected although one eye may be implicated earlier.

Visual field defect

The most common field defect is bitemporal hemianopia commencing in the lower quadrant and progressing to blindness.

Depending on the location and its growth there may be varied type of field defects.

Radiographic features

No radiographic evidence of damage to sellae turcica.

Endocrine disturbances

If the tumor grows to cause symptoms before adolescence then there is mal-development of the anterior lobe of pituitary producing hypopituitarism which can produce the following syndromes:

i. Fröhlich's syndrome: It is characterized by:

- Obesity around shoulders and hips
- Soft hairless skin
- Genital hypoplasia
- Impairment of dark adaptation
- Associated symptoms of increased sugar tolerance, polyuria, lethargy and narcolepsy.

ii. Lorain's type of infantilism: It is characterized by:

- Patient is small in height proportionate and attractive,
- Sexual underdevelopment
- Bright mentally

iii. Simmond's pituitary cachexia: It is characterized by:

- Looks aged prematurely due to dry and wrinkled skin,
- Loss of body hairs
- Vascular hypotension
- Amenorrhea or impotence due to gonadal deficiency

- General weakness with lethargy
- Mental apathy and psychoses

Symptoms due to pressure on neighbouring structures

Pressure on hypothalamus may produce adiposity, hypersomnia, polyuria and all other symptoms of involvement of the tuber cinereum.

Diagnosis

- Presence of constitutional signs of hypo-pituitarism.
- Bitemporal hemianopia, which starts in the lower quadrant.
- X-ray of pituitary fossa shows erosion of anterior and posterior clinoid processes. Fossa appears shallow and wide. Areas of calcification varying from small flecks to large masses.
- It is to be kept in mind that faint calcified shadow above the sellae may be due to an aneurysm of the internal carotid artery.

Management

Surgical excision.

5. SUPRASELLAR MENINGIOMA (Dural Endothelioma)

Suprasellar meningioma arises from the dura covering the circle of venous sinuses around the chiasmal sulcus and tuberculum sellae. Their pathology and nature is like that of *meningioma of sheath of optic nerve*. These are fibrous mulberry like slow growing tumors, slowly growing affecting adults.

These are rarely associated with endocrine disturbances or pressure symptoms on neighbouring hypothalamus.

Clinical Features and Management

Visual Loss

Due to the location of meningioma the optic nerves are involved earlier than the chiasma. As the tumor is not exactly placed in midline, so one nerve may get affected much earlier than the other by pressure therefore, may result in descending optic atrophy. The visual loss in one eye may occur much earlier than in the other eye.

Field Defect

Characteristic field defect is slow deterioration in the ipsilateral field and central scotoma in the other. Usually, central field defect merges with peripheral indentation producing an expanding sector defect in the visual field.

Optic Nerve

Optic neuritis is of common occurrence. Papilledema is rare.

X-ray Pituitary Fossa

In early stage there are no changes shown by X-ray. Later there is depression and atrophy of clinoid processes.

Management

Surgical removal of the tumor.

6. GLIOMA OF THE CHIASMA

Primary tumors of the chiasma are rare. Glioma is the most common tumor among primary tumors of the chiasma. Glioma of the optic nerve may extend backwards to chiasma and through the chiasma to hypothalamus. The glioma may be shared between the chiasma and optic tracts. Glioma occurs predominantly in children between 12 to 14 years of age. Visual symptoms for long period. Visual field defects are bitemporal hemianopia but frequently bizarre, irregular. Fundus often shows some degree of optic atrophy.

Diagnosis

Age: Glioma affects young children. Tumor of optic nerve with typical bitemporal hemianopia must be suspected for glioma of chiasma.

X-ray pituitary fossa: X-ray shows a characteristic deformity of sellae that is J-shaped gourd-like shadow. There is often destruction of sellae.

Management

Surgery is the only choice. The alternative therapy is radiation.

7. CHIASMAL NEURITIS

Chiasmal neuritis is neuritis of chiasma or tracts.

It is caused by the following:
- Multiple sclerosis
- Neuromyelitis of Devic's.

The onset is sudden and usually accompanied by headache and blurred vision. It can cause retrobulbar neuritis in that case fundus will show papillitis or optic atrophy.

Bilateral field defects are there though it may not be the typical bitemporal hemianopia.

Management

Systemic steroid is only choice and that too for long-time.

8. CHIASMAL ARACHNOIDITIS (CHIASMAL SYNDROME)

Etiology

It occurs commonly between 30 to 40 years of age.

It can be caused by trauma or infection.

Trauma: Traumatic basilar meningitis sets up local adhesive inflammation as it does in spine.

Infection can occur in three ways:
- As part of general hematogenous infection like tubercular or syphilitic meningitis
- As part of cerebral infection such as encephalitis
- Lymphatic spread from sinuses or nasopharynx
- Multiple sclerosis
- Rheumatic fevers
- Tendency of the arachnoid to continue as adhesive sclerosis long after the infection has become inactive or controlled
- Incidence of chiasmal arachnoiditis is not uncommon.

Pathology

The subarachnoid space below and anterior to the chiasma expands to cisterna chiasmaticus. Infections ususally start from here. The fine structure of arachnoid is transformed into a highly cellular dense membrane adhering to dura on outside and to pia on inside. It sets up interstitial neuritis or constricts the nerves or occlude the blood supply that leads to manifestation of optic atrophy.

On exploration there were inflammatory adhesions compressing the chiasma and the nerves. The field defects arise due to arachnoidal adhesions around the chiasma. The site and pressure by adhesions vary greatly, therefore the field changes also vary accordingly.

Clinical Features and Management
Visual loss

Vision is lost gradually over years or even suddenly. It may affect one eye or both the eyes. The visual acuity may vary from nearly normal to blindness.

Ophthalmoscopy

Fundus may be normal or may show slight hyperemia or pallor.

Optic atrophy is late manifestation.

Field defects
- Most common field defect is scotoma that is often bilateral and usually central, paracentral or cecocentral
- Bitemporal hemianopia
- Binasal hemianopia
- Concentric contraction of the peripheral field.

Management
- Systemic steroids to control infection and prevent adhesive process of arachnoid in form of adhesions and bands.
- Surgery to break the adhesions to retrieve chiasma from pressure.
- The fields show improvement after breaking the adhesions by surgery.
- It is difficult to decide which case should be taken for surgery and when surgery is risky.

9. SUPRACLINOID ANEURYSMS (ANEURYSM OF INTERNAL CAROTID ARTERY)

Supraclinoid aneurysms arise from carotid after this artery has pierced the dura. These appear at bifurcations of large vessels:

- At the origin of the ophthalmic artery just as the carotid is emerging from cavernous sinus on the lateral side of the anterior clinoid process.
- At the bifurcation of the internal carotid artery (Fig. 1.6).
- At the point where the anterior cerebrals join the anterior communicating arteries.

Aneurysm from any of these is likely to compress the optic nerve, chiasma or the optic tract.

Clinical Features and Management

- Symptoms appear during the phase of active expansion of aneurysm. Symptoms are intense headache, disturbance of vision, changes in the visual field of varying nature, usually a central scotoma.
- Aneurysm of internal carotid presses on the outer side of the angle of junction of nerve and chiasma.
- Characteristic field defect is epsilateral nasal hemianopia with partial temporal hemianopia in the other eye progressing to ipsilateral blindness with contralateral temporal hemianopia (Fig. 1.7).

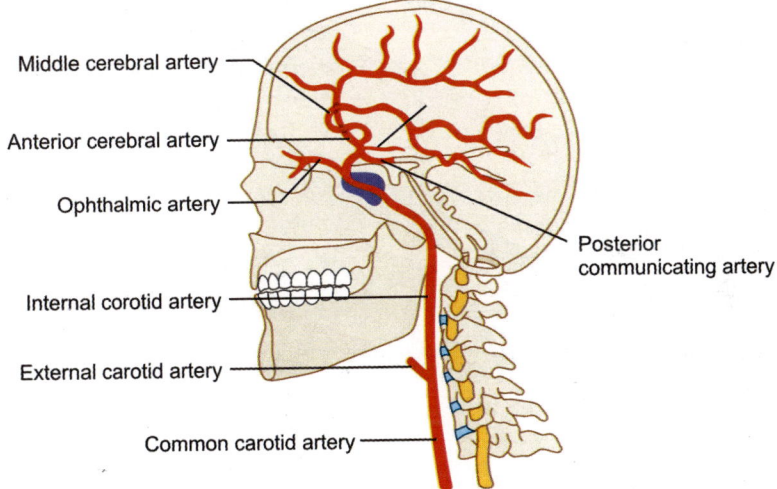

Fig. 1.6: Common carotid artery and its branches

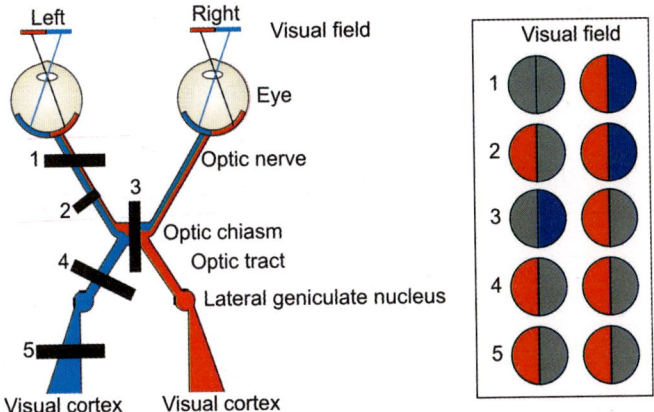

Fig. 1.7: Optic pathway with field defects

Management

Treatment is under the domain of neurologist. Refer the case to neurologist.

10. VISUAL FIELD DEFECTS IN CHIASMAL LESIONS

Though the nerve fibre pattern of the chiasma is constant yet there are other factors which must be taken into account in interpretation of the visual field changes due to chiasmal lesions (Fig. 1.8).

Factors which influence the field defects:

- Normal variation in the position of the chiasma, prefixed (with short optic nerves), in the middle position and post fixed (with long optic nerves).
- Normal variation in the bony structure of chiasmal area.
- Close relationship of chiasma with the following: Circle of Willis, pituitary body, pituitary stalk, third ventricle, tuberculum sellae and sphenoid ridge.
- Pressure on the chiasma at different points and from different directions.
- Direct or indirect pressure on the chiasma by neighbouring structures.

- Chiasma being pressed by a structure on one side directly and also being pressed by opposite structure indirectly.

From clinical point of view it shall be better if we discuss the chiasmal field defects according to specific lesions.

1. Infrachiasmatic Lesions

The most important infrachiasmatic lesion is the pituitary adenoma. The field defects vary depending on whether the chiasma is prefixed, in middle position or post-fixed.

- Typical visual field defect is a symmetrical bitemporal hemianopia of either the scotomatous or nonscotomatous type.
- Scotomatous type of bitemporal hemianopia indicates a rapid growth of tumor or prefixed chiasma with pressure on the posterior angle of chiasma or both the factorsthe rapid growth and pressure at the posterior angle.
- Symmetrical bitemporal hemianopia due to median chiasmal pressure from below occurs in the following sequence. The first field affected is in upper temporal quadrant followed by lower temporal

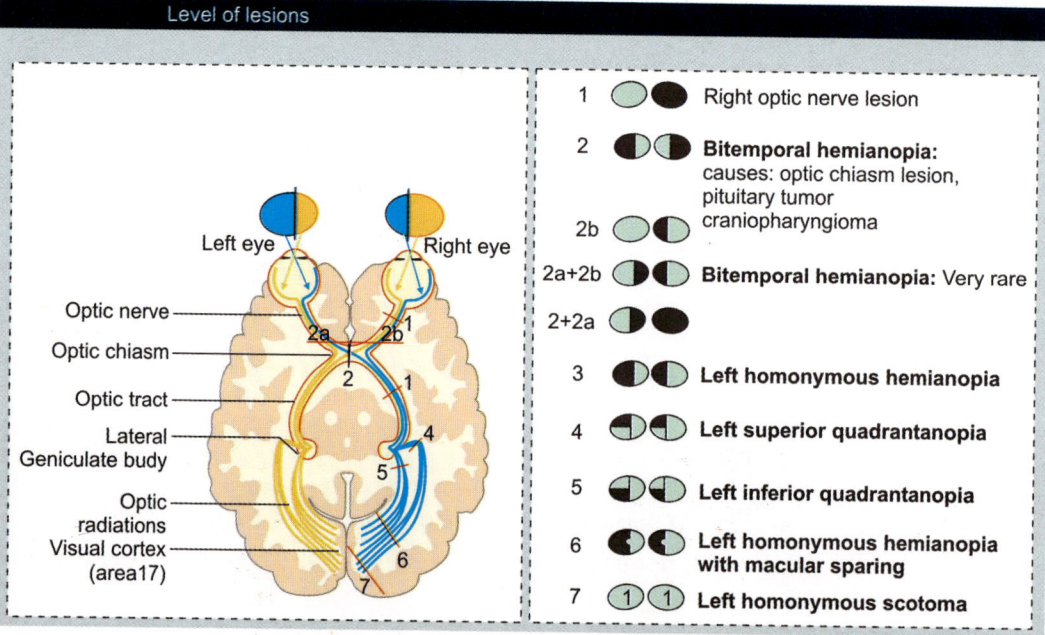

Fig.1.8: Visual fields in chiasmal lesions

quadrants. At this stage—the hemianopic field defect may remain static for some time before progressing to involve the lower nasal quadrant and finally the upper nasal quadrant.

Thus, it is seen that the progress of the field defect is typically clockwise in the right eye and anticlockwise in the left eye.

2. Suprachiasmatic Lesions

The typical field defect produced by the suprachiasmatic lesion is bitemporal hemianopia.

- In this case the first field affected is lower temporal quadrant followed by upper temporal quadrant thereafter the upper nasal quadrant and finally the lower nasal quadrant.
- Suprachiasmatic lesions may occur at two different locations and therefore the field defects shall vary.

i. Anterosupreior Lesions

- Most common lesion which affects the antero-superior part of the chiasma is meningioma.
- Meningioma may arise from olfactory groove, the tuberculum sellae or the lesser wing of the sphenoid bone.
- Other lesions are glioma and meningioma of the frontal lobe, aneurysm of the anterior cerebral arteries or the anterior communicating artery.

Meningioma of olfactory groove

- It is of common occurrence.
- It arises in the midline and extends straight backwards into the anterior chiasmal angle therefore the field defect is bitemporal hemianopia that begins in the lower temporal quadrant.
- Its eccentric growth will give rise to asymmetric field defect.

Meningioma of tuberculum sellae

- It arises close to the chiasma and causes pressure on its anterior angle therefore the field defect is bitemporal hemianopia that begins in the lower temporal quadrant.
- Its eccentric growth will give rise to asymmetric field defect.

Meningioma of the lesser wing of the sphenoid bone

- It arises lateral to the chiasma therefore the field defect is irregular and asymmetrical from chiasmal compression.
- Scotoma on the side of lesion is common field defect with or without hemianopic characteristics.
- Midline tumor will give rise to bi-temporal hemianopic field defect that is more advanced on one side.

Meningioma or glioma of the frontal lobe

- Tumor of frontal lobe is likely to compress one optic nerve on the side of tumor and may extend posteriorly to compress the chiasma from above.
- Field defect is asymmetric.
- Foster-Kennedy syndrome-denotes optic atrophy on the side of lesion and papilledema on the other side is the classic symptom of the frontal lobe tumor.

ii. Posterosuperior Lesions

- Most common lesions are craniopharyngioma and dilation of third ventricle.

Craniopharyngioma

- Typical field defect is bitemporal hemianopia that begins in the lower temporal quadrant.
- Field defect is not consistent due to its erratic growth.
- Central scotoma is frequent and occurs early.

Dilation of the third ventricle

- It can occur in the cerebellar tumor, acoustic neuroma, pinealoma and tumor of fourth ventricle.
- Field defect is due to uniform midline pressure against the posterior border of the chiasma from above.
- Earliest field defect is bilateral inferior quadrant scotoma that later becomes bitemporal hemianopic field defect.

iii. Perichiasmatic Lesions

- Perichiasmatic lesion is chiasmal archnoiditis.
- Supraclinoid aneurysm (aneurysm of the internal carotid artery).

iv. *Intrachiasmatic Lesions*

The common intrachiasmatic lesions are glioma of the chiasma and chiasmal neuritis.

Glioma of the chiasma

It grows erratically within the chiasma superiorly or inferiorly.

These may extend to invade the optic nerve or optic tracts. Therefore, the field changes shall vary greatly from scotomas to hemianopia.

The field changes are irregular and asymmetric.

Chiasmal Neuritis

- Most common cause for chiasmal neuritis is multiple sclerosis. The common field defect is bilateral central scotoma. *If the bilateral central scotomas show hemianopic characteristics then it is suggestive of chiasmal neuritis.* It helps to differentiate the chiasmal neuritis from ordinary bilateral retrobulbar neuritis and tobacco amblyopia.
- Other causes are neuromyelitis optica and sphenoidal or ethmoidal sinusitis.

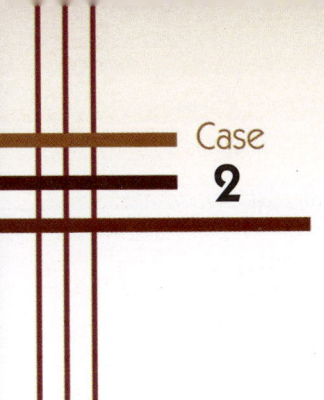

Ophthalmoplegia

An adult male attends ophthalmic clinic with complaint of mild pain in the right eye associated with diplopia, drooping of the lid and restriction of the eye movements particularly outwards. These symptoms appeared following recent attack of influenza with high fever for three days. Now, there is some diminution of vision also. Ocular examination shows ptosis with involvement of sixth and third cranial nerves.

Diagnosis: Ophthalmoplegia

OPHTHALMOPLEGIA

Opthalmoplegia is a malady in which there is paresis of ocular muscles.

Ophthalmoplegia is of various types with varied etiological factors.

It can be:

- Congenital or acquired
- External or internal
- Total or partial
- Unilateral or bilateral.

Ophthalmoplegia can be associated with:

- Pain in the affected eye or eyes
- Dim or normal visual acuity
- Varied systemic diseases like diabetes, hypertension, and arteriosclerosis
- Ophthalmoplegia can occur due to any lesion in the nerve nucleus, nerve trunk or the muscle itself.

Each case of ophthalmoplegia needs thorough history, clinical examination, clinical investigation to arrive at diagnosis.

Types of Ophthalmoplegia

1. External Ophthalmoplegia

It is a condition in which only extraocular muscles are involved (Fig. 2.1).

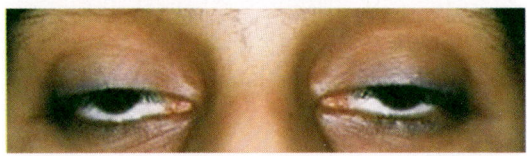

Fig. 2.1: Chronic progressive external ophthalmoplegia

When all the extraocular muscles are affected then it is known as *complete external ophthalmoplegia*.

When few muscles are affected then it is known as *incomplete or partial external ophthalmoplegia* (Fig. 2.2).

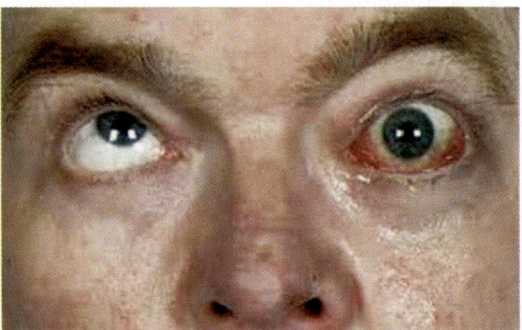

Fig. 2.2: Left eye ophthamoplegia

2. Internal Ophthalmoplegia

It is a condition in which only intraocular muscles are paralyzed.

3. Total Ophthalmoplegia

It is a condition in which all the extraocular and intraocular muscles are paralyzed.

Clinical Examination

History

- Time of onset and duration of ophthalmoplegia
- Is it since birth or acquired later in life
- Trauma or fever prior to onset of ophthalmoplegia
- Recent viral fever like cold, measles or mumps
- Metabolic disorder like diabetes or hypertension
- Endocrine disorder like thyrotoxicosis
- Associated headache indicating migraine
- Addiction to alcohol or drugs
- Associated weakness with exertion
- Difficulty in chewing the food
- Associated pain in the eye
- Drooping of one or both upper eyelid
- Diplopia.

Visual Acuity

Record the visual acuity in each eye separately and with both the eyes open. Correct the refractive error if any. If the visual acuity does not come to normal then investigate for the loss of vision.

Ocular Movements

There may be restriction of movements of the eye in one direction or more than one direction or there may be complete restriction with very little movement on effort.

Note down the presence or absence of movements so that the movements of the eye subsequently can be compared with the previous record. This will help to assess the progress and prognosis.

Pupillary Reaction

- Test the direct and consensual light reflex carefully.
- An ill-sustained pupillary reaction helps to clinch the diagnosis.
- Normal reacting pupil helps to exclude certain diseases.

Lid Movement

- Test for lid movements
- Look for ptosis
- Even insignificant ptosis helps to clinch the diagnosis.

Ophthalmoscopy

- Look especially for any change in the colour of optic disk.
- Pale colour or temporal pallor should be viewed with suspicion.
- Any changes indicating hypertension, arteriosclerosis or diabetes.

Laboratory Investigations

- Total blood picture
- Blood sugar—fasting and postprandial
- VDRL test
- RH factor
- Urine examination.

Clinical Investigations

- X-ray orbit, optic foramen and sphenoidal fissure
- CT Scan
- MRI
- Ultrasonography.

Etiological Classification

1. Congenital ophthalmoplegia

- Hereditary ophthalmoplegia
- Progressive congenital ophthalmoplegia.

2. Acquired ophthalmoplegia

Infections

- Encephalitis
- Acute cranial polyneuritis
- Orbital cellulitis
- Cavernous sinus thrombophlebitis.

Vascular

- Arteriosclerosis
- Aneurysm
- Hemorrhages and thrombosis
- Giant cell arteritis.

Myogenic

- Myasthenia gravis
- Myotonica dystrophy
- Myositis.

Neoplastic

Tumors and cysts of orbit
Nasopharyngeal tumor.

Metabolic

Thiamine deficiency
Diabetes
Thyrotoxicosis.

Traumatic

Trauma to the orbit
Fracture at base of skull
Trauma to midbrain.

Recurrent

Ophthalmic migraine

Exogenous

Barbiturates
Alcohol.

Common Causes of Bilateral Total Ophthalmoplegia

Encephalitis
Syphilis
Tumors of midbrain
Multiple sclerosis
Trauma.

Common Causes of External Ophthalmoplegia

Diabetes mellitus
Thyrotoxicosis
Myasthenia gravis
Orbital apex syndrome
Sphenoidal fissure syndrome.

Common Causes of Painful Ophthalmoplegia

Diabetes mellitus
Pseudotumor of orbit
Orbital periostitis
Sphenoidal fissure syndrome

Orbital apex syndrome
Collier's sphenoidal palsy
Tolosa-Hunt syndrome
Orbital abscess
Nasopharyngeal tumor.

Common Causes of Transient Ophthalmoplegia

Multiple sclerosis
Ophthalmic migraine
Recurrent oculomotor palsy
Hypertension
Arteriosclerosis
Diabetes
Collier's sphenoidal palsy.

CLINICAL FEATURES AND MANAGEMENT

1. Congenital external ophthalmoplegia
2. Congenital total ophthalmoplegia
3. Bilateral acquired complete external ophthalmoplegia
4. Bilateral acquired total ophthalmoplegia
5. Unilateral ophthalmoplegia of varying degree
6. Ophthalmoplegia due to nasopharyngeal carcinoma
7. Orbital apex syndrome
8. Collier's sphenoidal palsy
9. Sphenoidal fissure syndrome
10. Pseudotumor of the orbit
11. Tolosa-Hunt syndrome
12. Hypophyseosphenoidal syndrome
13. Petrosphenoidal syndrome
14. Recurrent oculomotor palsy.

1. CONGENITAL EXTERNAL OPHTHALMOPLEGIA

External ophthalmoplegia is the term applied to a condition in which all the extraocular muscles are paralyzed. Complete external ophthalmoplegia is a rare condition. It is common that some movement may be elicited when an effort is made to follow a moving object. In some cases a limited movement of the eyeball may occur in all the directions. An external ophthalmoplegia without ptosis is exceptional.

2. CONGENITAL TOTAL OPHTHALMOPLEGIA

Total ophthalmoplegia is a rare malady in that all the extra- and intraocular muscles are paralyzed. There is ptosis, immobility of the eyes and unreactive pupil to light and accommodation.

3. BILATERAL ACQUIRED COMPLETE EXTERNAL OPHTHALMOPLEGIA

An acquired bilateral and complete external ophthalmoplegia occurs due to catastrophic vascular or inflammatory lesion in the midbrain.

Vascular lesions

- Aneurysm
- Hemorrhage and thrombosis

Inflammatory lesions

- Encephalitis
- Acute cranial polyneuritis.

4. BILATERAL ACQUIRED TOTAL OPHTHALMOPLEGIA

An acquired bilateral total ophthalmoplegia is a rare malady involving pupillary and extraocular muscles.

Etiological factors

- **Aneurysm**: Suprasellar or intracavernous
- **Pituitary apoplexy**: Sudden enlargement of pituitary tumor.

5. UNILATERAL OPHTHALMOPLEGIA OF VARYING DEGREE

It manifests in the following four syndromes:
- Orbital apex syndrome
- Sphenoidal fissure syndrome
- Hypophyseosphenoidal syndrome
- Petrosphenoidal syndrome.

6. OPHTHALMOPLEGIA DUE TO NASOPHARYNGEAL CARCINOMA

The tumor may spread extracranially into the orbit from the pterygopalatine fossa. It may reach orbital apex from intracranial cavity through the superior orbital fissure. Thus, its spread gives rise to the 'syndrome of orbital apex' and 'syndrome of sphenoidal fissure'.

Spread of tumor from intracranial cavity shall affect the extraocular muscles earlier then the occurrence of proptosis.

Spread of tumor extracranially into the orbit shall show signs of muscle paresis and proptosis simultaneously.

Sometimes the tumor may invade the base of skull in the region of sphenoidal sinus and posterior ethmoidal air cells resulting in 'hypophyseosphenoidal syndrome'.

Petrosphenoidal syndrome is seen characteristically when nasopharyngeal carcinoma arises in relation to the fossa of rosenmuller with infiltration of peritubal region (eustachian tube) resulting in condition known as 'triad of Trotter' that is characterized by:

- Ipsilateral deafness
- Temporofacial neuralgia
- Palatal paresis.

The tumor rarely spreads through the eustachian tube or by its destruction. As a general rule the nasopharyngeal carcinoma spreads from the nasopharynx within the planes of the pahryngeal fascia surrounding the eustachian tube to pass towards the petrosphenoidal region with possibility of reaching the sphenoidal fissure and cavernous sinus region. Thus, it is liable to involve the VI cranial nerve at the apex of the petrous temporal bone, III nerve at the sphenobasilar suture at the base of the skull, V nerve in the region of gasserian ganglion and IV and II cranial nerves also.

From the above description, it is clear that acquired ophthalmoplegia can occur due to spread of nasopharngeal carcinoma, giving rise to four syndromes:

- Orbital apex syndrome
- Sphenoidal fissure syndrome
- Hypophyseosphenoidal syndrome
- Petrosphenoidal syndrome.

The 'triad of Jacod' is constituted by the following three syndromes:

- Orbital syndrome (orbital apex and sphenoidal syndrome)
- Hypophyseosphenoidal syndrome
- Petrosphenoidal syndrome

7. ORBITAL APEX SYNDROME (POSTERIOR OSTEOPERIOSTITIS)

It occurs due to inflammation, tumor or trauma in the region of orbital apex. There is axial proptosis, edema of the lids and chemosis of the conjunctiva all of which are common signs of any acute orbital inflammation.

The syndrome of orbital apex is associated with the 'triad of sensory-motor ophthalmoplegia'.

Immobile globe with internal ophthalmoplegia that is total ophthalmoplegia due to involvement of the oculomotor, trochlear and abducens nerves.

Anesthesia often associated with neuralgic pains in the area of distribution of the first division of the trigeminal nerve and sometimes even the area covered by second division also. Pain may precede the paralysis of ocular muscles.

Amaurosis due to post neuritic or post-papilledematous optic atrophy. Treat the cause. Short course of systemic steroids is beneficial.

8. COLLIER'S SPHENOIDAL PALSY

It is characterized by transient periostitis of the sphenoidal fissure inducing ocular motor paresis and frequently trigeminal anesthesia and neuralgia.

It affects at any age from puberty onwards.

It is comparable to Bell's palsy because it also arises from exposure to cold or sinusitis or without any obvious causative factor.

The malady commences with pain in the orbit, proptosis and progressive involvement of nerves passing through the superior orbital fissure follows—VI, IVth, first division of Vth, IIIrd, and second division of Vth in that order.

It may ultimately present as a case of total ophthalmoplegia with anesthesia in the area of distribution of first and second division of Vth nerve along with neuralgia.

Sometimes, it may show only involvement of VIth nerve alone.

Recovery is rule within few weeks to few months.

Course of systemic steroid helps in early recovery.

9. SPHENOIDAL FISSURE SYNDROME

It is characterized by:

- Total ophthalmoplegia—there is complete paralysis of extraocular and intraocular muscles,
- Anesthesia and neuralgia along the distribution of first and second division of the trigeminal nerve, and
- In this syndrome, there is no involvement of optic nerve. It can be caused by variety of factors such as, tumor of sphenoid bone, syphilis, trauma, encysted hematoma, pansinusitis and occlusion of superior ophthalmic vein.

10. PSEUDOTUMOR OF ORBIT (IDIOPATHIC ORBITAL INFLAMMATORY DISEASE)

It affects people in their middle age. It is usually a unilateral disease. Its onset is sudden. Patient complains of pain in the eye which is soon associated with lid edema, chemosis and congestion of the conjunctiva. There is proptosis with limitation of ocular movements without any inflammatory signs. It may resolve and may have attacks of intermittent episodes of acute activity. Often there is fibrosis of the orbital tissue resulting in a 'frozen orbit' which is associated with visual loss and ptosis. Computerized tomography scanning shows the enlargement of muscles and thickening of the sclera.

Ultrasonography demonstrates sonolucency (edema) posterior to the globe. The area behind the globe appears in the form of a square and not in the usual W-shaped optic nerve area.

11. TOLOSA-HUNT SYNDROME

It is characterized by:

- Unilateral ophthalmoplegia of varying degree due to paresis of ocular nerves.
- Pain which may be periorbital or hemicranial.
- Sensory loss along the first division of trigeminal nerve.
- Pupil may show abnormal reaction.
- Responds well to systemic steroids.

It is to be differentiated from orbital apex syndrome, superior orbital fissure syndrome and inflammatory process of cavernous sinus.

12. HYPOPHYSEOSPHENOIDAL SYNDROME

Ophthalmoplegia due to this syndrome is produced by a lesion in the base of skull, in the region of sphenoidal and posterior ethmoidal sinuses.

It is frequently associated with destruction of dorsum sella.

Sometimes the nasopharyngeal carcinoma invades the base of skull in the region of sphenoidal and posterior ethmoidal sinuses resulting in this syndrome.

Sometimes, there is involvement of the III, IV, VI nerves, in the region of the cavernous sinus giving rise to bilateral ophthalmoplegia.

Implications of V nerve shall give rise to neuroparalytic keratitis. Sometimes optic chiasma may be affected producing typical visual field defects.

13. PETROSPHENOIDAL SYNDROME

This syndrome arises when a nasopharyngeal carcinoma spreads from nasopharynx within the planes of the pharyngeal fascia surrounding the eustachian tube to pass towards the petrosphenoidal region with invasion of the sphenoidal fissure and cavernous sinus.

It is characterized by:

- Ophthalmoplegia
- Severe neuralgia due to involvement of Vth nerve
- Loss of vision due to involvement of IInd nerve
- Horner's syndrome due to involvement of sympathetic nerve supply.

Involvement of IXth, Xth, XIth, XIIth cranial nerves due to posterior spread of the nasopharyngeal carcinoma.

Usually, the VIIth and VIIIth cranial nerves escape due to protection by the temporal bone.

14. RECURRENT OCULOMOTOR PALSY

It can be unilateral or bilateral most commonly occurring between the age of 50 to 60 years. The common causes are sinusitis, diabetes, ophthalmic migraine, cranial neuritis, multiple sclerosis, arteriosclerosis, periostitis of apex of orbit, rheumatism and scleritis. It responds to topical and systemic course of steroid.

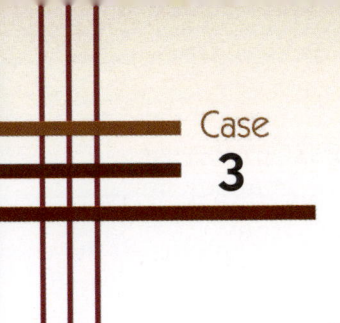

Sixth Nerve
Paralysis—Right Eye

Middle aged person attends the ophthalmic clinic with complaint of double vision since this morning. The double vision is particularly on looking towards the right side. Ocular examination shows limitation of the eye movements of the right eye on outward movement. All other ocular movements are normal.

Diagnosis: Right lateral rectus paralysis

ABDUCENS SIXTH NERVE

Paralysis of the sixth (abducens) cranial nerve can occur due to any lesion at any point in its long course from the nucleus to the lateral rectus muscle (Fig. 3.1). It shall not be out of way to discuss here in short the origin and course and the relations of the sixth nerve during its course to have better understanding of the malady.

Origin

The abducens nerve arises by seven or eight rootlets. The rootlets emerge between the lower border of the pons and the lateral part of the pyramid. The rootlets join to form one nerve at a varying distance from the origin.

COURSE AND RELATIONS OF SIXTH NERVE

1. AT THE ORIGIN

There is a distance of about 1 cm between the origins of two abducens nerves. The basilar artery formed by the two vertebrals lie between these two abducens nerves. The facial nerve arise lateral to the abducent nerve. Because of this proximity of the sixth (abducent) and seventh (facial) nerves any lesion at the level of the pons results in the involvement of both the nerves.

2. IN THE POSTERIOR CRANIAL FOSSA

Sixth nerve moves forward, upward and slightly laterally between the pons and the occipital bone. After about 15 mm it pierces the dura lateral to the dorsum sellae. The nerve runs upwards on the back of the petrous temporal bone near its apex. At the sharp upper border of the petrous bone

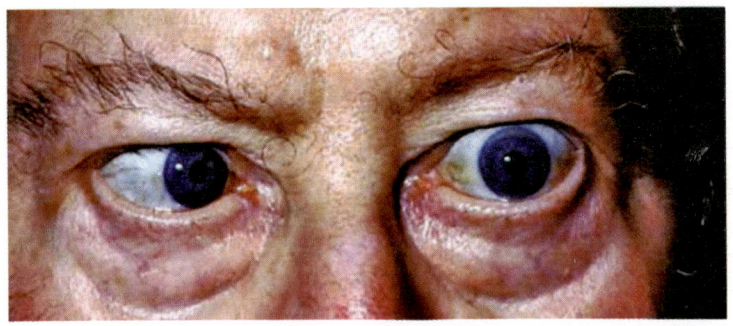

Fig. 3.1: Abducens nerve paralysis—right eye

the nerve bends forward at right angle under petrosphenoidal ligament to enter the cavernous sinus. Because of the bending of the nerve at right angle at the sharp upper border of the petrous bone it is most frequently involved nerve in cases with rise of intracranial pressure due to any cause, tumor or inflammation.

Sixth nerve also gets frequently involved due to traction or pressure by the anterior inferior cerebellar and internal auditory arteries as they cross the nerve at right angles and often lie ventral to the nerve. The nerve comes under pressure between the arteries and the pons.

3. IN THE CAVERNOUS SINUS

Sixth nerve runs almost horizontally forward, below and lateral to the internal carotid artery. The carotid is surrounded by the sympathetic plexus.

Cranial nerves from above downwards in the lateral wall of the sinus (Fig. 3.2):

- Oculomotor (third) nerve both the divisions
- Trochlear (fourth) nerve
- Ophthalmic division of the trigeminal (fifth) nerve
- Maxillary division of the trigeminal (fifth) nerve.

Gasserian (trigeminal) ganglion and the temporal lobe of the brain are immediate lateral relations of the cavernous sinus.

In cavernous sinus thrombosis all these cranial nerves are involved and the sixth nerve gets involved earliest. With the involvement of the second eye the earliest sign again is the paresis of the sixth nerve.

Involvement of the sixth nerve is due to its course along the internal carotid artery.

4. IN THE SUPERIOR ORBITAL FISSURE

Sixth nerve passes through the superior orbital fissure within the annulus. The lateral rectus muscle takes its origin from both the margins of the fissure.

Sixth nerve in its course through the superior orbital fissure can get involved in the following:

- Superior orbital fissure syndrome,
- Collier's sphenoidal palsy.

In both the conditions it is the sixth nerve that gets paralyzed earliest. In Collier's sphenoidal palsy the paresis of the sixth nerve may be the only presenting sign.

5. IN THE ORBIT

In the orbit the sixth nerve enters the medial (ocular) surface of the lateral rectus muscle

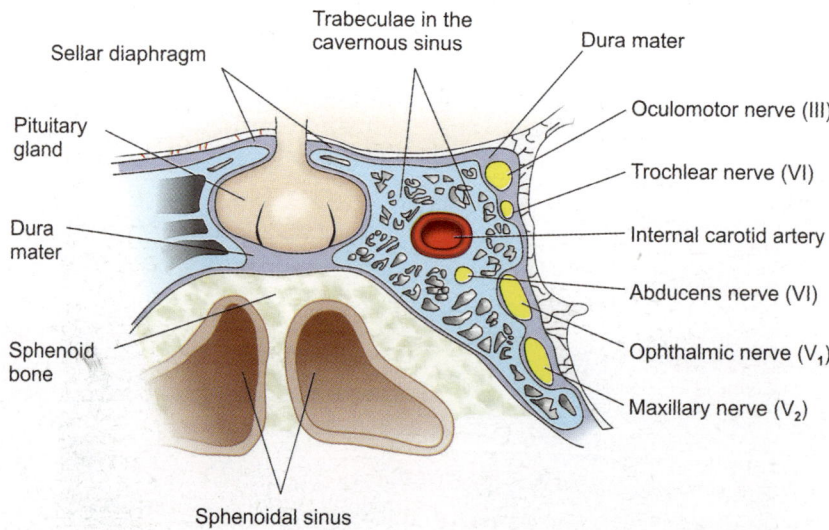

Fig. 3.2: Structures passing through the cavernous sinus and its lateral wall

just behind its middle portion after branching in three or four branches.

Thus, the sixth nerve gets involved in any inflammatory or space occupying lesion of the orbit easily.

The limitation of ocular movement is usually first noticed in the outward direction.

NUCLEUS OF THE ABDUCENS NERVE

The nucleus of the sixth nerve is small spherical mass which consists of large multipolar cells. It lies close to midline in the segmental portion of the pons.

The nucleus of the sixth nerve can be affected in viral encephalitis, space occupying lesion of brain, hemorrhagic and thrombotic lesions in the midbrain.

With the discussion of the long course of the sixth nerve, it can be concluded that this sixth nerve can get involved by various lesions at various sites. Thus, the paresis of the sixth nerve as such has no localizing value unless associated with other specific signs and symptoms pertaining to that structures or structures in close association with the sixth nerve.

Etiology

Most common factors:
- Collier's sphenoidal palsy
- Superior orbital fissure syndrome (Fig. 3.3)
- Arteriosclerosis
- Diabetes
- Hypertension
- Trauma.

Clinical Features

1. Primary Position

The right lateral rectus muscle is an abductor therefore in its primary position the right eye appears deviated inwards due to over action of the right medial rectus which is an ipsilateral antagonist of the right lateral rectus.

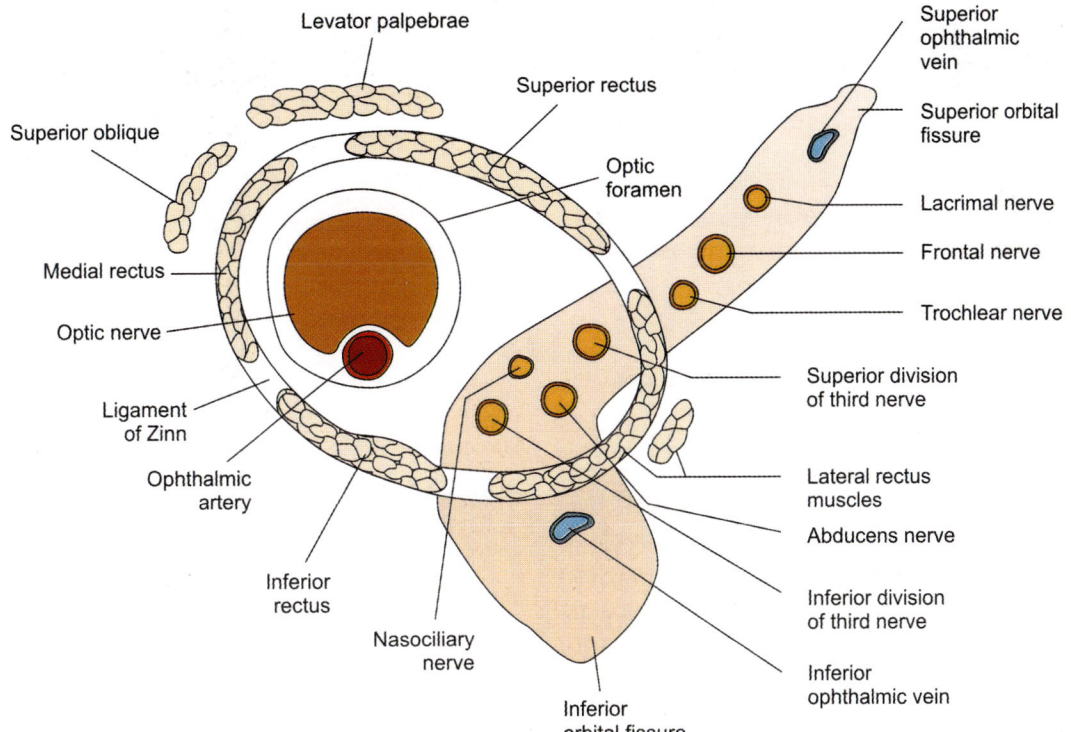

Fig. 3.3: Structure passing through orbital fissure

The secondary deviation of the normal left eye during fixation with the paralyzed right eye is also convergence due to over-action of the left medial rectus (the contra-lateral synergist) and secondary under-action of the left lateral rectus (the antagonist of the contralateral synergist Fig. 3.4).

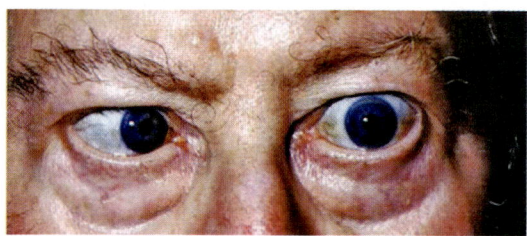

Fig. 3.4: Sixth nerve palsy—right eye

Note the following points:

- **In recent case:** The secondary deviation is greater than the primary deviation, ii.
- **Later:** Due to contractures developing in the ipsilateral antagonist the secondary deviation becomes equal to primary deviation of the eye. At this stage the strabismus appears to be concomitant and not paralytic.
- **Still later:** With further development of contractures of contralateral synergist with secondary underaction of the antagonist of the contralateral synergist the primary deviation increases. Therefore, the paralyzed eye fails to reach the midline even with an effort.

2. Esotropia

There is esotropia in the primary gaze.

3. Limitation of the Abduction

The restriction of outward movement may be very slight. Conduct examination carefully and compare with the outward movement of the opposite eye.

All other ocular movements are normal.

4. Compensatory Head Posture

Compensatory head posture is usually mild rotation of the face towards the side of paralysis that is right side in this case.

This rotation of face towards the field of action of paralyzed muscle is to over-come the diplopia.

5. Field of Binocular Fixation

Field of binocular fixation shows constriction towards the paralyzed side.

6. Diplopia

Diplopia is uncrossed and increases towards the paralyzed side. Displacement of the image is horizontal.

There is slight vertical displacement of the image when the paralyzed eye is in position of adduction (inwards).

Slight vertical displacement of image in adduction (inwards) is due to increased effect of the oblique muscles in the adduction (inward) position.

7. Hess Chart

Hess charting shows the following:

- Shrinkage away from the direction of action of the right lateral rectus muscle.
- Enlargement towards the direction of action of right medial rectus muscle (ipsilateral antagonist) and of the left medial rectus muscle (the contralateral synergist).
- Shrinkage away from the direction of action of the left lateral rectus muscle (the antagonist of the contralateral synergist).

8. False Projection

False projection is outwards to the paralyzed side.

Clinical Investigations

- Visual acuity is normal unless there is involvement of the optic nerve.
- Limitation of the abduction
- Uncrossed diplopia
- Hess charting shows shrinkage of the field.

Laboratory Investigations

- Blood sugar fasting and post-prandial
- Total and differential count.

Other Investigations

- General and systemic examination to exclude, any septic focus, arteriosclerosis and hypertension.
- X-ray paranasal sinus will be helpful.

Management

- Treat the cause
- Systemic broad spectrum antibiotic and Steroids
- General line of treatment with vitamins and minerals
- Most of the cases show improvement with the above treatment as the common cause for an isolated sixth nerve palsy is in the Orbit-Collier's sphenoidal palsy which is like Bell's palsy.

Some cases do take long-time but all show improvement in the ocular movement and the distressing symptom of diplopia.

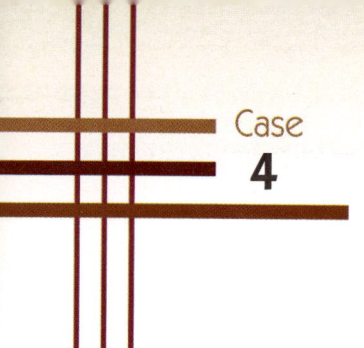

Carotid-Cavernous Aneurysm

Arteriovenous aneurysm in the cavernous sinus is the most common cause of pulsating proptosis (Fig. 4.1). Arteriovenous fistula is usually in the cavernous sinus thus it is better known as *carotid-cavernous aneurysm/fistula* (Fig. 4.2).

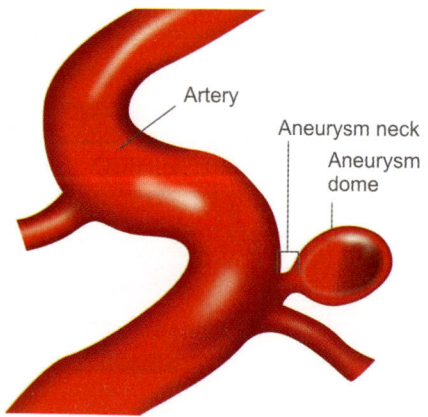

Fig. 4.1: Diagram showing aneurysm

CORTICOCAVERNOUS FISTULA

Occurs in two conditions:

1. TRAUMATIC COMMUNICATION

- Traumatic cases occur frequently in males and covers about 80% of total cases.
- Cases are mostly associated with fracture of the base of skull of which 70% cases have fracture involving the body of sphenoid.
- Rupture of the carotid artery occurs in the cavernous sinus.
- Trauma need not cause rupture immediately but may damage the arterial wall so that saccular aneurysm is formed and that gives way.

2. SPONTANEOUS COMMUNICATION

- Spontaneous communication between carotid and cavernous develops as a

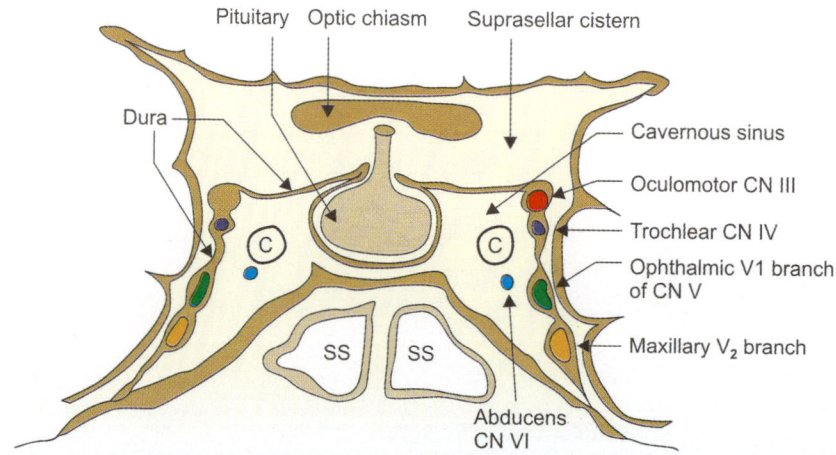

Fig. 4.2: Diagram showing relations of cavernous sinus

result of the bursting of aneurysm of carotid or weakness of vessel wall both of which have congenital factor.

- Seen also as familial occurrence.
- Spontaneous communication is more common in females.
- Aneurysm of carotid in the cavernous may eventually give way most commonly in the conditions of atheroma, arteriosclerosis or hypertension.

MECHANISM OF PULSATING PROPTOSIS

Due to rupture of carotid artery in the cavernous sinus there is a direct escape of arterial blood under high pressure into the cavernous sinus. It causes increase in the venous pressure and the flow of the blood is reversed mostly into the ophthalmic veins. The enormously dilated tortuous ophthalmic veins result in stasis, edema of the orbit and proptosis with transmission of pulse to the orbital contents, lids and the globe synchronous with the systolic beat.

Clinical Features

- In traumatic cases the onset of symptoms may be sudden on recovering consciousness from head injury with marked unilateral pulsating proptosis, a swishing noise in the head, pain and visual loss. In many cases of trauma the onset may be gradual. Trauma causing damage to arterial wall to form aneurysm that gives way at later stage.
- In spontaneous cases which are associated with congenital weakness of the arterial wall or aneurysm the onset of symptoms are sudden. Patient feels a crash in his head with violent pain and characteristic bruit. The pulsating proptosis appears soon with symptoms of vomiting and vertigo.

The patient may become unconscious and even die.

- *Proptosis* is rapidly progressive, axial and pulsatile with engorged ophthalmic veins at upper and inner angle of the orbit.
- *Pulsation* may be accompanied by a bruit which may be heard with stethoscope over the temple or directly over the eye. The sound may be soft or shrill. Sometimes the patient complains of listening a sound like—rushing of water, water fall, roar of a train or rumble of mill.
- *Cardinal symptoms of pulsation* with bruit are increased on stooping and decreased or disappear on compression of carotid on affected side.
- *Other symptoms* are chemosis of conjunctiva, swelling of lids, full veins, signs of anterior segment ischemia, vascular changes in the fundus in the form of microaneurysms, intraretinal and superficial hemorrhages.
- *Anterior segment ischemic* changes include: filamentary keratitis, bullous keratopathy, neovascularization of cornea, aqueous flare, iris atrophy and paralysis of pupillary muscles.
- Raised intraocular pressure that may lead to blindness.
- Involvement of cranial—third, fourth, fifth, and sixth nerves in the wall of cavernous sinus, is of common occurrence with diplopia as an early symptom.

Prognosis

The course and prognosis is not good. In some cases there is spontaneous recovery due to thrombosis in the aneurysm spreading towards the orbit. There may be a sudden and immediate death with rupture of cavernous sinus and cerebral hemorrhage.

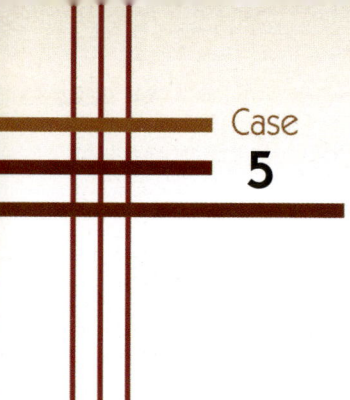

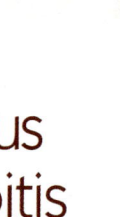

Cavernous Sinus Thrombophlebitis

A cavernous sinus thrombophlebitis is a grave malady with very high mortality rate if not diagnosed and treated early and energetically (Figs 5.1 and 5.2). Delay in treatment may save the life of patient but is likely to be blind either due to damage to cornea or optic atrophy.

ETIOLOGY

a. *Infection by venous stream*: The most common etiological factor is the spread of infection by venous stream from neighbouring infected structures; such as tonsilitis, sinusitis, mastoiditis, squeezing pimple on the nose or stye, dental abscess, hordeolum and furuncle on the face (eyebrow, cheek, lip, nose or chin).
b. *Orbital cellulitis*
c. *Trauma*
d. *Ostitis of orbital bones.*

CLINICAL FEATURES

There is acute onset with rapid presentation of symptoms. At first the malady is unilateral but sooner or later it spreads to other eye through the circular sinus then the symptoms are bilateral.

a. *Pain*: Patient complains of severe pain over the eye and forehead on the affected side with hyperesthesia over the area of distribution of ophthalmic division of the fifth nerve. At first it is on one side which may become bilateral with the spread of infection to opposite side.

b. *Edema of lids*: The lids are edematous, swollen, and hard with woody feeling. The veins over the lids are dilated. The skin appears red and tense. It is difficult to examine the eye without the help of lid retractor.

Anatomy of the cavernous sinus

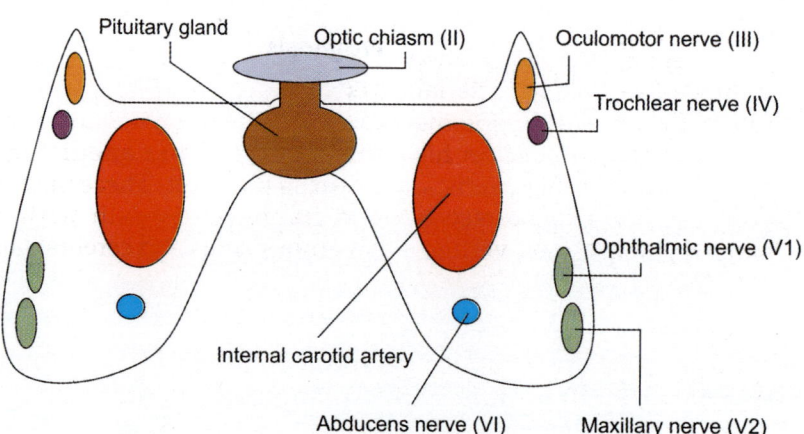

Fig. 5.1: Structures passing through cavernous sinus

c. *Conjunctival congestion and chemosis*: The conjunctiva is markedly congested with severe chemosis. The lower conjunctiva may protrude out through closed and swollen lids and may show signs of necrosis.

d. *Proptosis*: It develops rapidly and is axial and irreducible. Proptosis may be so marked as to endanger the cornea by exposure keratitis.

e. *Cornea*: There is corneal anesthesia with clouding and ulceration.

f. *Ophthalmoplegia*: It may be of varying degree. Ultimately the globe becomes completely immobile due to involvement of third, fourth and sixth cranial nerves in the cavernous sinus wall.

g. *Fundus changes*: Ophthalmoscopy may show retinal venous engorgement, hemorrhages and mild papilledema. Later ophthalmoscopy may show postneuritic or papilledematous optic atrophy.

h. *Visual acuity*: There is a loss of visual acuity of varying degree. It is due to papillitis, macular edema or ischemic optic neuropathy.

i. *General symptoms*: Patient is extremely ill will high swinging temperature, rigors and rapid pulse. Presence of neck rigidity with severe pain in the head is indicative of intracranial spread.

Complications

The infection from cavernous may spread anteriorly to cause orbital cellulitis

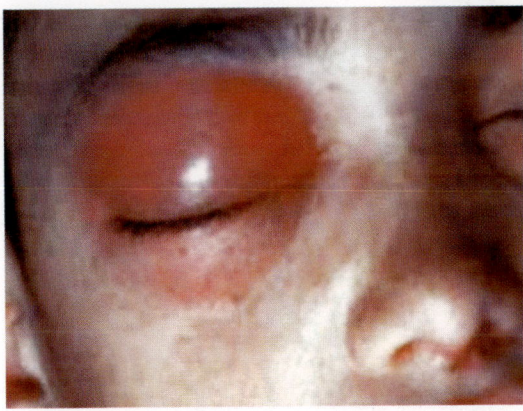

Fig. 5.2: Cavernous sinus thrombophlebitis

and orbital abscess. It can extend intracranially to cause cerebral and cerebellar abscesses.

Pathogenesis

The signs and symptoms are mainly due to stagnation of venous return.

Ophthalmoplegia is due to involvement of cranial nerves in the cavernous sinus wall.

Proptosis is due to stagnation and infection of the orbital tissue.

Corneal anesthesia is due to involvement of fifth nerve.

Management

- Antibiotic along with steroid drugs are the sheet anchor of treatment. These drugs should be given in massive doses and intravenously.
- All kind of supportive therapy.
- Protection of cornea is important.

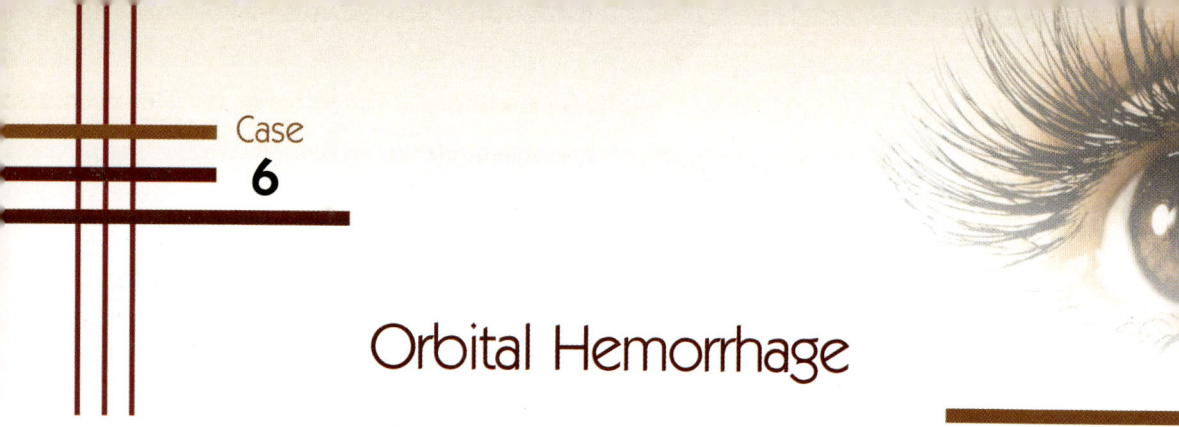

Case

6

Orbital Hemorrhage

Orbital hemorrhage can be conveniently divided into three factors:

i. Due to system diseases
ii. Due to venous congestion
iii. Due to direct trauma.

1. DUE TO SYSTEMIC DISEASES

Hemorrhagic Diathesis

a. *Hemophilia*

Orbital hemorrhage may occur spontaneously, after mild trauma or surgical interference. There is an acute proptosis which may even endanger the cornea. It may result in visual loss due to compression of optic nerve. There is tendency for recurrences.

b. *Scurvy*

Bleeding is due to defect in the cement substance between the endothelial cells of the capillaries. This in turn is due to lack of ascorbic acid that is common in children. It can be treated by systemic administration of vitamin C as medication and in diet. As a rule bleeding in the orbit occurs between the bony roof of the orbit and the periostium thereby pushing the globe forwards, downwards, and outwards. If the proptosis is sufficient to threaten the cornea then the hemorrhage should be cleared by a sub-periosteal approach. The blood may seep through the orbital fascia, presenting as a purple line around the orbital margin or ecchymosis.

Arterial Disease

General arterial diseases such as arterio-scelrosis, hypertension and renal diseases may cause recurrent orbital hemorrhage.

Local arterial disease like aneurysm or varix may result in orbital hemorrhage.

Vasomotor Instability

Orbital hemorrhage has been observed in females at the time of climacteric and with attacks of neuroparalytic migraine.

2. DUE TO VENOUS CONGESTION

Venous congestion is not an usual cause. Orbital hemorrhage and proptosis results from thoracic compression or strangulation. Other causes can be violent and spasmodic cough, lifting of heavy weight or any condition wherein there is tendency for venous congestion for a long-time.

3. DUE TO DIRECT TRAUMA

Orbital hemorrhage due to direct trauma is common cause for proptosis.

• It is seen following a retrobulbar injection prior to surgery. In these cases the proptosis is acute and may be extreme in case the surgeon does not apply a firm pressure over the eyeball with closed lids. A firm pressure and thereafter a firm bandage for 24 hours is immediate treatment. It checks bleeding and controls proptosis as well.

• Orbital hemorrhage can result due to breaking of arterial branches by contre-coup trauma. Usually, the bleeding is mild limited to subconjunctival hemorrhage in the lower and outer quadrant with diplopia and mydriasis.

• Any injury which may cause fracture or penetrating injury can result in orbital hemorrhage (Fig. 6.1).

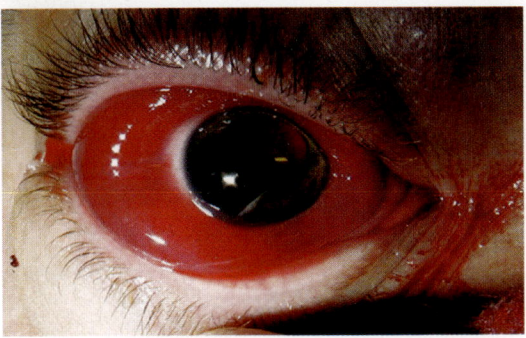

Fig. 6.1: Orbital hemorrhage

Clinical Features

- An acute orbital hemorrhage produces acute proptosis.
- Proptosis is irreducible, axial or eccentric with no ocular movements.
- Lids are swollen, puffy with ecchymosis.
- Pupil is dilated with no reaction.
- Fundus shows papilledema and retinal hemorrhages.
- Intraocular pressure is very high.

Complications

- Exposure keratitis
- Pressure effect may lead to optic atrophy.
- Acute radiating pain in the orbit. It is usually associated with vomiting due to *trigeminovagal stimulation* which excites an oculogastric reflex. It may also excite an *oculocardiac reflex* thereby slowing the heart rate.

Management

- The orbital hemorrhage absorbs slowly in few weeks or months.
- Treat the case as per its cause.
- Rest and ice compresses are helpful.
- Some cases may need evacuation of blood by aspiration or incision.
- Some cases may need orbital decompression.
- Broad spectrum antibiotic systemically and locally shall help prevent infection of hematoma.

Lid Nodule Carcinoma

Patient attends the ophthalmic clinic with complain of nodule on the lid margin for a long-time. There is no pain or tenderness. He has come for cosmetic purpose. Ocular examination shows lid squamous cell carcinoma.

Diagnosis: Lid squamous cell carcinoma

Carcinoma is a common cutaneous form of malignant tumor affecting the lid. It occurs in two forms—squamous cell carcinoma (Fig. 7.1) and basal cell carcinoma (Fig. 7.2).

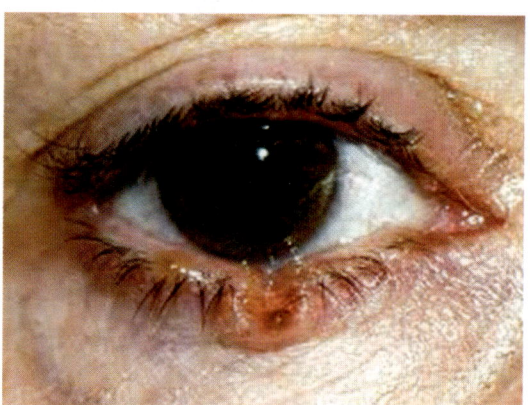

Fig. 7.2: Basal cell carcinoma

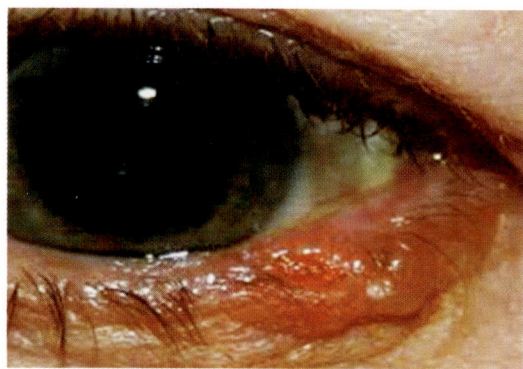

Fig. 7.1: Squamous cell carcinoma

Incidence

Age

Carcinoma affects people commonly between the age of 50 to 70 years.

Sex

There is a slight predominance of males. Some authors have found no difference between the sexes.

Race

Carcinoma is disease of caucasians. Basal cell carcinoma is the most common tumor of the skin in white races.

Duration and Size

Patient usually presents after a long duration of years due to its slow growth with no symptoms. In most cases the carcinoma is discovered during a routine clinical examination of the eye. The size of the lesion is related to the duration. It can vary from 5 mm to 2 cm.

Site of Lesion

Most common site for the basal cell carcinoma is the skin near the margin of the lower lid nearer to inner canthus.

Most common site for squamous cell carcinoma is the skin of the upper lid nearer to outer canthus. The lower lid is affected much more than the upper lid.

Etiology

Etiology is not known. But about 30% of cases have an association of trauma or irritation as trigger.

Factors Acting as Trigger

- Chronic blepharitis
- Eczema
- Injuries
- Squeezing of black heads or pimples
- Actinic radiation—bright sunlight with low humidity
- Old cicatrix
- Lupus vulgaris
- Senile papillomata
- Senile keratosis
- Precancerous dermatosis
- Cases with high sebaceous glands
- Exposure to radiation

1. SQUAMOUS CELL CARCINOMA

Cilinically

- Squamous cell carcinoma commences (Fig. 7.1) as small hard indurated nodule that after few months show erosions and fissures with crust and eventually manifests as ulcer.
- At this stage of ulceration the base of the ulcer is always sharply defined, indurated, hyperemic with hard edges which are undermined.
- If not taken care at this stage and allowed to grow then there is a local extension. It extends gradually and slowly eating away skin, connective tissue, cartilage, periosteum and bone covering large area on the face.
- There is a foul smell with a large fungating ulcer like crater.
- To begin with there is no pain and that is why there is delay on the part of patient to get treated. Later with involvement of the infraorbital or supraorbital nerves there is a marked pain which may become excruciating.
- Regional lymph nodes are involved due to secondary infection and in some cases from cancerous extension.

- There is progressive cachexia and emaciation.
- Eventually the patient dies after a long period of suffering due to hemorrhage, meningitis, general exhaustion, septicemia or cachexia.

Histopathology

- There is an epidermal invasion of the corium with epithelial arrangement of cells in groups.
- In a section the downgrowth appears as finger-like claws extending from the main mass and in continuity with it.
- Squamous cell carcinoma is characterized by cellular processes which retain the structure of the epidermis—peripherally there are cylindrical cells, internal to these are large prickle cells and in centre there are squamous cells, all arranged in compressed, laminated masses, staining strongly eosinophilic with acid dyes known as 'cell nests' or 'epithelial pearls'.
- If these cells are clearly differntiated then the tumor is less malignant than if there is no clear differentiation of cells.

Metastasis

- Metastasize by perineural lymphatics so the regional lymph nodes are first affected.
- Metastasis from upper lid drains into the preauricular lymph nodes.
- Metastasis from lower lid drains into the submaxillary lymph nodes.

2. BASAL CELL CARCINOMA (RODENT ULCER: BASILOMA)

Clinically

- Basal cell carcinoma (Fig. 7.2) is the most common tumor of the eyelids much more common than the squamous cell carcinoma.
- It occurs exclusively on hair-bearing skin and commences as a small, shiny, translucent nodule or a scaly patch.
- After few months this nodule or patch shows ulcer in the central area and the

periphery shows appearance of small pearly satellite nodules.

- Eventually ulcer is formed with indurated base and raised nodular edge. It grows slowly and painlessly extending superficially and deeply eating away the surrounding structures manifesting as large crater as seen in squamous cell carcinoma.

Histopathology

- Microscopic picture differs from that of squamous cell carcinoma.
- Processes grow downwards at uniform level and show expanded club-shaped form.
- Cells are basophilic with scanty cytoplasm.
- All the cells are of one type, i.e. basal cells of the epidermis. There are no prickle cells, no cell nests, no cornification and no eosin staining of cells.

Metastasis

- Extremely rare.
- Lymph nodes are affected due to secondary infection.

Diagnosis of Carcinoma

- Any small nodule eroded or crusted or persistent ulcer in the lids particularly in person above 40 years of age should always arouse suspicion for a carcinoma until it is unproved otherwise.
- Absence of lymphadenopathy further confirms the suspicion.
- Biopsy through full thickness of the lesion.

Management of Carcinoma

- In early stage—surgery with complete excision of the lesion.
- Later when a large area has been involved then excision and or radiation may be employed.
- Excision should always be wide covering healthy tissue.
- Microscopy of the excised tissue is essential to confirm whether complete excision has been achieved or not. If not, then radiotherapy must be employed.
- Basal cell carcinoma is more sensitive than the squamous cell carcinoma for radiotherapy.

Prognosis

- Prognosis is good with early complete excision that is confirmed by histopathology.
- Prognosis is poor in cases with involvement of large area with lymphadenopathy.
- Prognosis of squamous cell carcinoma is worse than that of basal cell carcinoma.
- Prognosis for upper lid carcinoma close to inner canthus is worse.

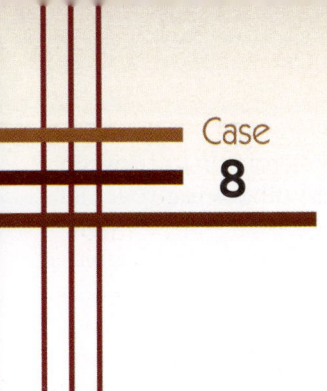

Keratic Precipitates

Patient enters the clinic with complain of blurred vision in his right eye since three months. The blurring of the vision was gradual. He has consulted opticians. There is no improvement in his vision with any glasses. No other complain or symptom.

On examination, the visual acuity in his right eye is 6/24, with blurring. The visual acuity in his left eye is 6/6, with clarity. External examination is normal. Pupil is reacting normally. Red reflex is not clear in his right eye.

Slit lamp shows keratic precipitates.

Diagnosis: Keratic precipitates.

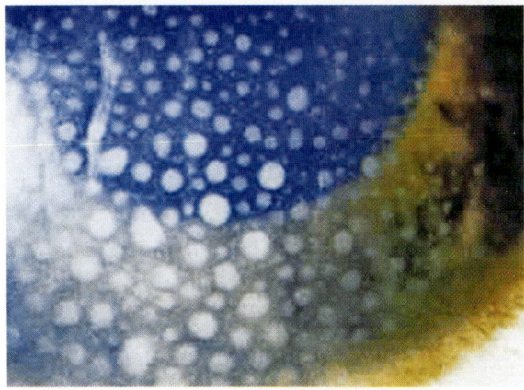

Fig. 8.1: Keratic precipitates—fresh white waxy

KERATIC PRECIPITATES

This is a condition in which there is deposition of material on the posterior corneal surface. Keratic precipitates are composed of macrophages, lymphocytes and plasma cells. The deposits on the corneal endothelium vary in size, colour, shape and distribution.

Clinical Features and Managment

Appearance of precipitates is preceded by edematous changes in the corneal endothelium.

Typically, the precipitates are seen in a triangular form in the lower part of the corneal endothelium. This peculiar distribution is due to convection currents in the aqueous humor.

Keratic precipitates are composed of chronic inflammatory cells—macrophages, lymphocytes and plasma cells.

Large sized keratic precipitates are typical of granulomatous-uveitis. In early stage these are white and waxy (Fig. 8.1)

in appearance and later stage shows brown and crenated appearance (Fig. 8.2). These are composed of epitheloid cells and mononuclear macrophages.

Presence of keratic precipitates is suggestive of chronic cyclitis. Patient may not have any other symptom except low and blurred vision due to deposition of exudates on the posterior corneal surface. The blurred vision can also occur due to

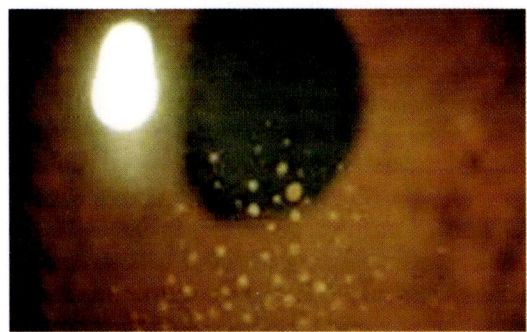

Fig. 8.2: Keratic precipitate old brown irregular

pouring of inflammatory cells and exudates in the vitreous.

Diagnosis

Keratic precipitates can be diagnosed easily with retroillumination method of slit lamp with retroillumination biomicroscopy.

Management

As the presence of keratic precipitates is pathognomonic for uveitis, therefore, treat the case as a case of uveitis, as follows:

• Course of systemic antibiotic.

• Course of systemic steroids in full dose and taper off gradually with the improvement in signs and symptoms.
• Topical instillation of steroid and antibiotic eyedrops, six times a day.
• Topical instillation of cycloplegic, atropine eyedrops twice a day to achieve full mydriasis and thereafter maintain it.
• Investigate the case to find out the causative factor for uveitis.
• Regular check-up with slit lamp is essential to know the progress of the malady.

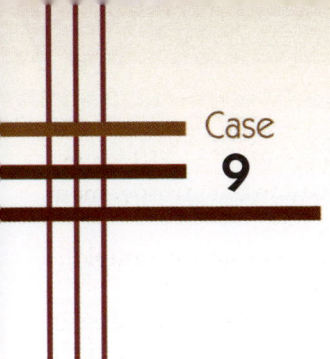

Rubeosis Iridis

Patient presents with no vision in his left eye since last ten years or so. There was no history of any symptom except gradual loss of vision in left eye. Now, the eye is painful.

Ocular examination shows intense circumciliary congestion.

Slit lamp shows rubeosis iridis left eye.

There is no perception of light. The eye feels stony hard.

Diagnosis: Rubeosis iridis

Rubeosis Iridis

- Rubeosis iridis is a condition of neovascularization of the iris, angle of the anterior chamber and the trabecular meshwork (Fig. 9.1).
- Most common causes for rubeosis iridis are central retinal vein occlusion and diabetic retinopathy.
- Pathogenesis involved is retinal ischemia.

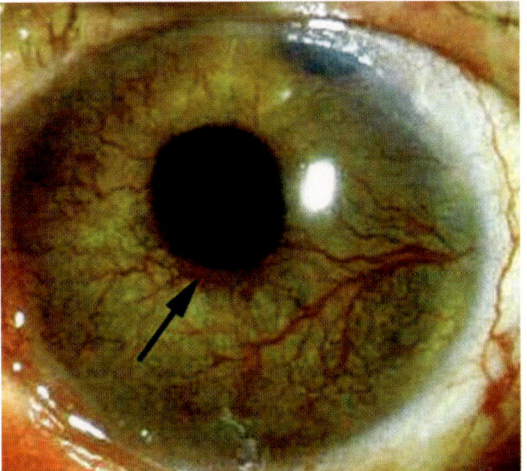

Fig. 9.1: Rubeosis iridis

- Neovascular glaucoma is the most common complication of rubeosis iridis.

Etiological Factors

- Central retinal vein occlusion
- Diabetic retinopathy
- Eales's disease (retinal perivasculitis)
- Coat's disease
- Central retinal artery occlusion
- Retinal detachment undiagnosed or untreated
- Giant cell arteritis
- Atrophic bulbi due to any cause.

Pathogenesis

- Rubeosis iridis starts as dilated capillary tufts at the pupillary margin and thereafter progresses towards the angle of the anterior chamber.
- Sometimes, there is a dilated vessel at the collarette which is joined by the capillary network from the pupillary margin.
- At this stage, the intraocular pressure is normal and the rubeosis iridis may regress either spontaneously or due to treatment of retinal ischemia.
- Treating the retina at this stage with panretinal photocoagulation may be successful in inducing regression of rubeosis iridis.
- New vessels on the iris continue to grow over and across the iris surface and join the circumferential ciliary body artery.
- New vessels then proliferate across the angle and invade the trabeculum. Also in this stage, there is formation of peripheral

anterior synechia which results in the rise of intraocular pressure.

- At this stage also, if the ischemic retina is treated with photocoagulation, then the hypoxic areas of the retina becomes anoxic. This will reduce or abolish formation of vasculogenic factor from the hypoxic retinal areas and results in regression of rubeosis iridis.
- Further stage is complete closure of the angle of the anterior chamber by formation and contraction of the fibrovascular tissue. The iris is pulled up over the whole of trabecular meshwork. The pupil is distorted.
- At this stage the eye is intensely congested with circumciliary congestion.
- Intense pain in the eye, which is unbearable.
- Patient himself may suggest excision the eye but desires relief from pain.
- Marked rise of intraocular pressure usually above 60 mmHg.
- Eyeball feels stony hard.

Clinical Investigations

1. Slit lamp shows new vessels formation on the iris.
2. Gonioscopy shows completely block of angle by the new vessels and iris with peripheral anterior synechia.
3. Fluorescein iris angiography shows rubeosis iridis seen by slit lamp.

Histopathology

It shows the lining of the capillaries with endothelial cells without a basement membrane. That is the how, the vessels bleed easily and cause hyphema even with trivial trauma to the eye.

Management

Pan-retinal photocoagulation helps to regress or stop the progress of rubeosis iridis.

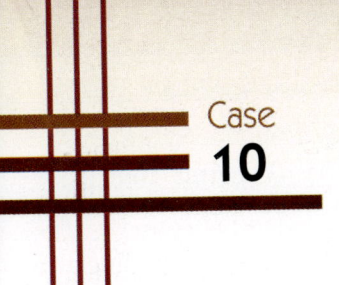

Traumatic Hyphema

Baby girl 9 years of age is brought to the ophthalmic clinic as an emergency case after being hit by the skipping rope while skipping at home, hitting her right eye. On ocular examination, there is mild congestion of the conjunctiva, lacrimation, discomfort, blurred vision and hyphema up to lower border of the pupil with a horizontal line.

Diagnosis: Traumatic hyphema with fluid blood

TRAUMATIC HYPHEMA

Clinical Examination

Test to Confirm About Fluidity of Hyphema

If the hyphema is fluid, then one can observe a horizontal line across the anterior chamber as the fluid always is in level (Fig. 10.1). Change the position of the head and the fluid blood moves and the horizontal line also changes accordingly. This confirms about the fluidity of the hyphema.

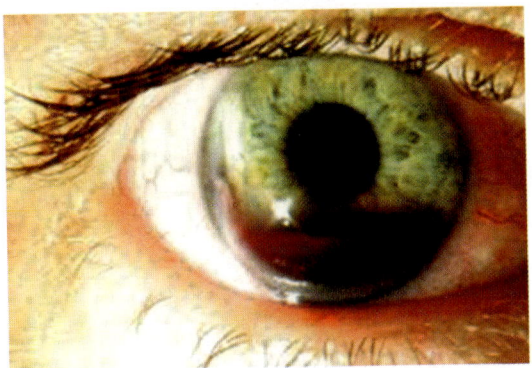

Fig. 10.1: Traumatic hyphema—horizontal line indicates fluid blood

In a case with clot of blood in the chamber there is no horizontal level. The upper border of the hyphema is irregularly convex upwards in the centre and sloping towards the periphery. It does not change the position with the change in the position of the head of the patient.

Slit Lamp Biomicroscopy

It shows early changes of blood staining in the cornea and sign of anterior uveitis in the form of synechia or keratic precipitates.

Tonometry

Rise of intraocular pressure favours blood staining of the cornea and uveitis, peripheral anterior synechia and optic atrophy. It is essential to keep or maintain the intraocular pressure below 25 mmHg to prevent blood staining of the cornea and optic atrophy.

If the intraocular pressure cannot be maintained even by adequate medical therapy then plan to evacuate the blood from the chamber soon without further delay. Surgical evacuation will prevent many unwanted complications which, most likely, cannot be treated effectively to prevent visual loss.

Ophthalmoscopy

Avoid active dilation of the pupil to prevent secondary hemorrhage. Any active dilation within 5 days of initial trauma is likely to disrupt the clot causing rebleeding from insured vessels. Ophthalmoscopy helps to observe early changes of optic atrophy due to raised intraocular pressure.

Gonioscopy

Gonioscopy should be performed in every case of traumatic hyphema after 10 to 15 days of initial injury when the hyphema has absorbed completely. Gonioscopy helps to exclude:

- Recession of the angle of anterior chamber
- Peripheral anterior synechia.

Clinical Features and Management

Hyphema occurs due to an injury to iris or ciliary body. The children are more prone to injury while playing. Hyphema may be small in amount or large filling the entire chamber and may remain fluid or become a clot during the very first day. If the hyphema is fluid and filling the chamber half or less then it shows horizontal line confirming the fluidity of the blood while blood clot in the chamber shows an irregular or convex line. There are more chances for fluid hyphema to get absorbed without causing rise of intraocular pressure. Hyphema in the form of blood clot in the chamber shall take long-time to absorb and is most likely to cause rise in the intraocular pressure.

Hyphema always induces anterior uveitis and can cause the following complications:

1. Secondary hemorrhage (rebleeding)
2. Secondary glaucoma due to block at the pupil and or at angle
3. Angle recession glaucoma
4. Hemolytic glaucoma
5. Ghost cell glaucoma
6. Peripheral anterior synechia
7. Optic atrophy
8. Blood staining of the cornea.

1. SECONDARY HEMORRHAGE (REBLEEDING)

- Secondary hemorrhage occurs when the hyphema is in the clot form and this clot of blood retracts causing injury to already injured vessels of iris.
- Secondary hemorrhage usually occurs during third to fifth day after the initial

trauma to the eye. If the healing has not been complete by this time then the retraction of the blood clot causes reopening of the injured vessel.

- Secondary hemorrhage is more difficult to treat reducing the visual prognosis.
- Secondary hemorrhage—rebleeding occurs in about one-third of cases.
- Secondary hemorrhage has no relation to the amount of blood in the anterior chamber.
- Any case of hyphema irrespective of amount should be treated with care and caution.
- To prevent secondary hemorrhage it is very essential to provide complete rest to the patient therefore the children with traumatic hyphema must be hospitalized to keep them out of activity which is not possible at home. Parents cannot ensure that their child will remain quiet without any activity at home.
- Parents must be made to understand the importance of re-bleeding and its complications with poor visual prognosis.

2. SECONDARY GLAUCOMA

Secondary glaucoma is directly related to two factors:

- *Amount of hyphema in the chamber.*
- *Type of blood (fluid or a clot) present in the chamber.*
  - The blood in the anterior chamber may remain fluid for long-time or may clot on the very first day.
  - If the hyphema is large even filling the anterior chamber to two-thirds or more, but is fluid in character, then there are all the chances for its quick absorption and no rise of intraocular pressure. Nursing the patient in a sitting position will clear the upper part of angle through which the aqueous will flow out helping the blood to absorb.
  - If the hyphema is large filling the anterior chamber to two-thirds or more and the clot has formed then it will take long-time for its absorption

and it is most likely to cause rise in the intraocular pressure. Rise in the intraocular pressure is due to block of the pupil and at the angle causing obstruction to circulation and outflow for aqueous. Such case needs evacuation of blood clot in the anterior chamber by surgery to prevent blood staining of the cornea with total visual loss. Delay is likely to induce peripheral anterior synechia that augments further rise in the intraocular pressure favouring blood staining of cornea.

– Hyphema in form of liquid or clot filling half or less than half of the anterior chamber is most likely to get absorbed without causing any rise of intraocular pressure as the pupil and angle both are not blocked with open circulation and outflow facility for aqueous.

– There are two routes for absorption of blood from the anterior chambers— the trabecular meshwork and uveal tissue (iris and ciliary body). Most of the absorption occurs through the trabecular meshwork.

– The blood itself and its disintegrated products induce iritis therefore, steroids and cycloplegics are must to prevent occurrence of synechia at the pupil and peripheral anterior synechia, jeopardizing circulation and outflow of the aqueous.

3. ANGLE RECESSION GLAUCOMA

- Angle recession occurs at the time of original injury.
- Angle recession is always due to contusion trauma to the eye.
- Contusional trauma causes tear of the ciliary body which results in the recession of the angle of the anterior chamber.
- Anterior chamber appears deep in that part.
- Small recession of the angle of anterior chamber may pass unnoticed as it does not show any obvious clinical finding or any rise of intraocular pressure.

- Large recession of the angle of the anterior chamber will show rise of intraocular pressure as there is obstruction to the outflow facility.
- Gonioscopy is mandatory in every case of hyphema to know the condition of the angle after the hyphema has absorbed.
- Quite often a case with recession of angle presents months after the original trauma with high intraocular pressure.
- Angle recession glaucoma is like open angle glaucoma.
- Angle recession glaucoma respond well to medical therapy.

4. HEMOLYTIC GLAUCOMA

Hemolytic glaucoma is the result of macrophage response incited by the disintegrated products of the blood in the anterior chamber.

Macrophages plug the pores of the trabecular meshwork causing obstruction to outflow facility of aqueous.

5. GHOST CELL GLAUCOMA

Ghost cell glaucoma is due to block of the trabecular meshwork by the rigid cell membrane of empty erythrocytes.

6. PERIPHERAL ANTERIOR SYNECHIA

- Presence of blood in the anterior chamber induces formation of peripheral anterior synechia.
- If the hyphema persists for more than 9 days one can expect formation of peripheral anterior synechia.
- Peripheral anterior synechia can be delayed by systemic administration of steroids for short duration.

7. OPTIC ATROPHY

- The high intraocular pressure causes decrease in the vascular perfusion in the optic nerve and retina resulting in decline in final visual acuity. Intraocular pressure above 35 mmHg even for 7–10 days can affect the vascular perfusion. Therefore, keep the intraocular pressure below 25 mmHg, by medical therapy.

- Avoid topical miotics to prevent constriction of pupil that favours pupil block and re-bleeding by dislodging clot.
- If the intraocular pressure cannot be maintained below 25 mmHg then it is better to plan surgical evacuation of blood.

8. BLOOD STAINING OF THE CORNEA

Blood staining of the cornea is one of the common complication of the traumatic hyphema (Fig. 10.2).

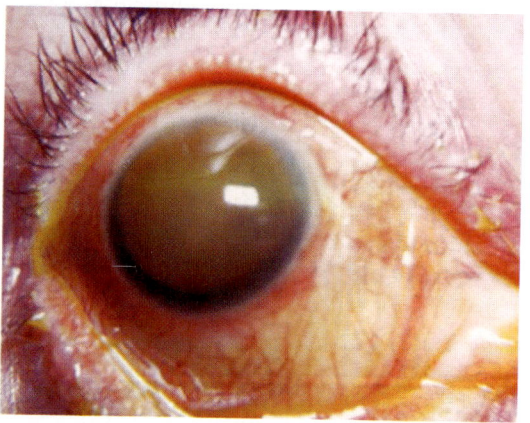

Fig. 10.2: Blood staining of cornea

Blood staining of the cornea is seen in the cases who have hyphema filling the anterior chamber more than half and the blood is in the clot form.

Rise in the intraocular pressure is pre-requisite for blood staining of the cornea. The rise in the intraocular pressure can occur due to the following factors: Block at the pupil, block at the angle, peripheral anterior synechia, associated iritis, disintegrated products of the blood plugging the pores of the trabecular meshwork and angle recession due to trauma.

There is no treatment once the cornea has become stained with blood. Prevention is the only choice available.

It can be achieved by topical instillation of steroids and cycloplegics and monitoring the intraocular pressure at regular intervals.

A slit lamp biomicroscopy shall help to diagnose blood staining early on its onset.

If there is any indication of blood staining then lower the intraocular pressure by intensive and adequate medical therapy and plan to evacuate hyphema surgically.

Clinically

Blood staining involves first the central part of the posterior corneal stroma seen only by slit lamp. Thereafter the blood staining spreads to cover the entire corneal stroma leaving only a small rim of clear cornea in the periphery.

Corneal stroma shows light brown to orange colour granules in the posterior corneal stroma.

These granules may extend to anterior corneal stroma in the course of time. The cornea itself appears red rusty brown in colour which later on changes to greenish yellow or grey in colour.

The blood stained eye gradually ends up as an atrophic bulbi.

It can become unbearably painful.

Cryopexy may help.

Some cases may need excision with fixing an artificial eyeball.

Management

Complete bedrest with hospitalization

The question is whether the patient of traumatic hyphema should be hospitalized or allowed to take treatment at home with visits to clinic for check-up everyday.

Eye is an important organ. How will it react to trauma is not definite as it differs with each case.

- We do not have any means to know the amount of thrust and force the eye has been subjected by trauma that may look very minor on its face value.
- Secondary hemorrhage occurs within 5 days of the initial trauma.
- Occurrence of secondary hemorrhage has no relation with the amount and type of hyphema.
- Even a slight trauma can cause secondary hemorrhage which gives poor visual prognosis.

- Keeping all the above mentioned factors in view it is advisable to hospitalize the patient as indoor patient to prevent the unwanted complication that affects severe visual loss.

- Even the most careful, educated and intelligent parents cannot ensure that the child will remain quiet without any active activity for all the first five days during which the chances of secondary hemorrhage are greatest.

- Even if the child is constantly under attendance of parents it is not sure that the transport of the child for recheck-up everyday shall not be the cause for secondary hemorrhage.

- Thus, in the interest of the patient and his visual recovery the child must be hospitalized. If not then the parents must be explained that even a slight trauma may lead to secondary hemorrhage. It is to be remembered that one-third cases develop secondary hemorrhage.

- Apart from the active activity and minor trauma there are other factors which can precipitate secondary hemorrhage. The most important factor is active dilation or constriction of the pupil by mydriatics and miotics. Active dilation of the pupil for examination of the posterior segment should be avoided. Active constriction of the pupil by miotics to treat the raised intraocular pressure should be avoided. Treat secondary glaucoma by timolol maleate and acetazolamide and osmotic agents.

- The view that the iris plays an important role in absorption of blood is not confirmed. Miotics shall dislodge the clot and induce irritative iritis.

- A moderate dilation of pupil with cycloplegic (atropine) is indicated to treat the associated uveitis. It does not cause active dilation of the pupil active dilation of the pupil is achieved by use of phenyl epinephrine along with cycloplegics especially used for examination of the posterior segment of the eye. Avoid it.

- A case of traumatic hyphema filling the anterior chamber with fluid blood needs nursing in sitting posture so that the blood gravitates leaving the upper part of the angle free for outflow. This position may not be maintained at home leading to rise of intraocular pressure.

- Thus to conclude, if the patient has hyphema up to 2 to 3 mm in the chamber or up to lower border of the pupil, or small clot, with pupil reacting normally, good red reflex, normal visual acuity, educated parents and can come for check-ups regularly, then one can allow the patient to be treated at home.

- If the case is having hyphema filling the entire chamber, the patient must be hospitalized irrespective of the nature of blood whether fluid or a clot.

- This patient is likely to develop raised intraocular pressure and all the associated complications of hyphema. The case will need a better nursing, check-up by slit lamp and tonometry twice a day, so that the blood staining and raised pressure can be diagnosed early and steps taken to prevent these by keeping the intraocular pressure well below 25 mmHg.

Cycloplegics

Use of cycloplegic is must in every case of hyphema irrespective of the amount and type of blood in the anterior chamber.

An active dilation of pupil by phenyl epinephrine and tropicamide to examine the posterior segment of the eye should be avoided for at least 10 days. An active dilation of the pupil can dislodge the clot and cause secondary hemorrhage.

The ideal choice for cycloplegia is instillation of atropine eye drops once or twice a day as per requirement in the case. Atropine causes effective and slow dilation of the pupil.

Steroids

Steroids are must in every case of hyphema for 5 to 7 days irrespective of the amount and the type of blood (fluid or a clot) in the anterior chamber. Topical instillation of steroids is not safe as it reduces the rate of aqueous outflow, therefore, it will reduce the rate of clearance of blood from the chamber through the trabecular meshwork.

Systemic steroids are safe and do not delay the rate of aqueous outflow. Systemic steroids reduce the chances of rebleeding. Thus, steroids given systemically for 5 to 7 days are safe and prevent complication of rebleeding which is common especially in children. There is no need to taper off the steroids and withdraw after 7 days.

Antiglaucoma Therapy

Secondary glaucoma occurs in the eye with hyphema filling the entire chamber and showing no signs of resolution.

Raised intraocular pressure above 35 mmHg for more than 5 to 7 days can be the cause for blood staining of the cornea and damage to the optic nerve by depriving it of its nutrition by vascular perfusion.

If the intraocular pressure is high then the aim of treatment is to keep it well below 25 mmHg.

Treat the glaucoma by instillation of timolol maleate eye drops: 0.5% twice daily.

If the intraocular pressure is still high then add systemic acetazolamide tablets for 5 to 7 days. With the resolution of hyphema the pressure will come down on its own.

Do not prescribe topical miotic as it causes active constriction of the pupil. Active constriction of the pupil may dislodge the clot and cause secondary hemorrhage. Topical miotic induces iritis due to irritation and pupillary block due to marked constriction of the pupil.

Surgical Evacuation of Hyphema

Most cases do not need surgical interference to clear the hyphema.

Surgical evacuation of blood is indicated if there is constant rise of intraocular pressure that may lead to blood staining of the cornea.

SUMMARY

This patient is baby girl 9 years of age so needs hospitalization for 7 days with complete bedrest.

Instil atropine eye drops once daily to moderately dilate the pupil.

Systemic steroid daily for 5–10 days or as per need.

Conduct slit lamp biomicroscopy daily to keep watch on the cornea and aqueous for any signs of uveitis and blood staining of the cornea.

Tonometry is not indicated and the child will also not allow tonometry without a struggle or anesthesia, both are more harmful for the final outcome and progress of a case.

If there is a suspicion for raised pressure, treat conservatively by timolol maleate eye drops for 5 to 7 days. It will not cause any harm though less formation of aqueous will delay clearance of blood from the chamber.

Younger the patient more important is the management, therefore, either hospitalization or complete rest at home is must and first requisite for proper treatment, progress and prognosis with good outcome of visual acuity.

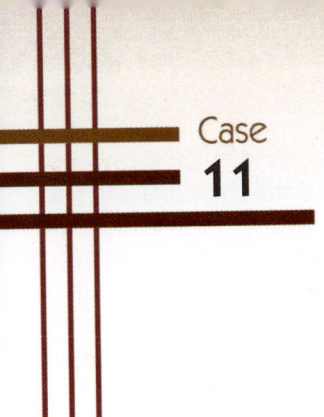
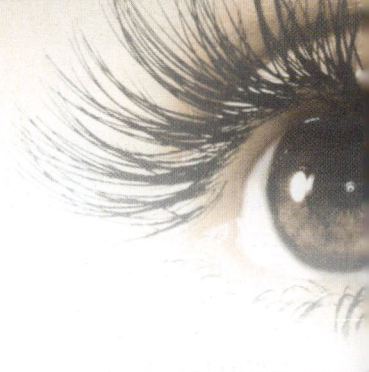

Case
11

Chemical Burn
Injury of the Eyes

Young female attends ophthalmic emergency with history of chemical being splashed in the eyes and face just an hour ago while working in laboratory as technician. She managed to wash her eyes and face immediately with plenty of water. She is feeling burning and photophobia. Ocular examination shows numerous spots of chemical burn on the skin of the face and lids. Lids are swollen. There is intense congestion of the conjunctiva with mild chemosis. The cornea shows erosion in the lower part that stains with fluorescein.

Diagnosis: Chemical injury of the eyes

CHEMICAL BURN INJURY OF THE EYES

Chemical injury of the one or both the eyes are not uncommon and may vary in severity from mild irritation to complete loss of the eye or eyes.

Most of the chemical injury is due to external contact with the chemical in the form of particles, powder, dust, liquid, gas, mist or vapour.

Systemic absorption of chemical can show its toxic effects on the visual pathway.

Systemic absorption occurs through the skin, lungs, and alimentary tract.

Incidence

1. Domestic Accidental Injury

Domestic accidents with chemicals are known to occur with the following:

• Ammonia
• Solvent
• Detergent
• Cosmetics
• Any chemical used in home.

2. Fog and Smog

Fog is minute droplets of water in the atmosphere. Fog is condensation of moisture around the minute particles present in the atmosphere.

Smog is combination of fog and industrial or automobile smoke consisting of gases and solid minute particles and causes irritative or allergic conjunctivitis and even keratoconjunctivitis.

3. Agricultural Chemical Injury

There are large number of chemicals used in the agriculture such as lime, superphosphates, ammonium phosphates, potassium sulphates, potassium chlorides, magnesium sulphates, and nitrates, etc. All these can damage the cornea by erosions, opacities and even perforation.

4. Laboratory Chemical Injury

Laboratory chemical injury usually involves eyes and face of students or technicians while working.

5. Industrial Chemical Injury

Chemical industries are source for large number of cases being injured at a time. Thus, chemical industry is hazard to public life and health. At the same time industry is required for growth and development. Protective measures adopted by industries shall help to reduce the number of cases getting injured and thereby disturbing the economics of family and nation.

6. Chemical Warfare

All the nations have become conscious about the hazards of chemical warfare. Therefore, now there is a ban on use of chemical warfare weapons.

7. Chemical Drugs

Chemical drugs such as silver nitrate, tincture of iodine, carbolic acid, calomel powder, skin ointment and many others are likely to injure the eye if not used carefully by the applicant or patient himself.

Mechanism of Chemical Injuries

The mechanism of chemical injury depends on many factors. The following factors will decide the type and severity of damage to the eye.

- Duration of contact
- Concentration of the chemical
- Solubility of the chemical
- Penetration of chemical in the tissue
- Form of chemical whether particle, liquid or gas
- Removal of chemical or neutralizing the chemical
- Reflex of the person to close the eyes.

Chemical in the form of a gas is in less concentration then liquid and particles.

Chemical in liquid form enters the eye before the person can react. Yet it can be washed off easily with plenty of water.

Chemical in form of particle may remain in contact with the eye tissue for long-time and its removal may be difficult or delayed.

An intelligent person will know the danger by the smell of the chemical and will react to it by moving away or washing the eyes immediately on feeling even mild irritation.

Blepharospasm will cause delay in washing the eye with water properly. Lacrimation is helpful in washing out the chemical.

Absence of pain is dangerous as observed with solutions of ammonium hydroxide or sulphur dioxide.

CLINICAL FEATURES AND MANAGEMENT

1. Sulphuric acid burn injury
2. Amonium hydroxide burn injury
3. Calcium hydroxide burn injury

1. SULPHURIC ACID BURN INJURY

An employee working with automobile battery dealer attends the clinic with history of acid drops spill in his eyes accidentally. He has washed his eyes immediately with water. He complains of burning sensation with redness and white spot on his cornea (Fig. 11.1).

Ocular examination shows conjunctival congestion, more in the lower fornix and one small white spot about 2 mm in the lower part of the cornea with sharp margins.

Diagnosis: Sulphuric acid burn of the cornea.

Sulphuric Acid Burn of Cornea and Face

Acid burns, whether the acid is inorganic or organic, produces almost a similar clinical

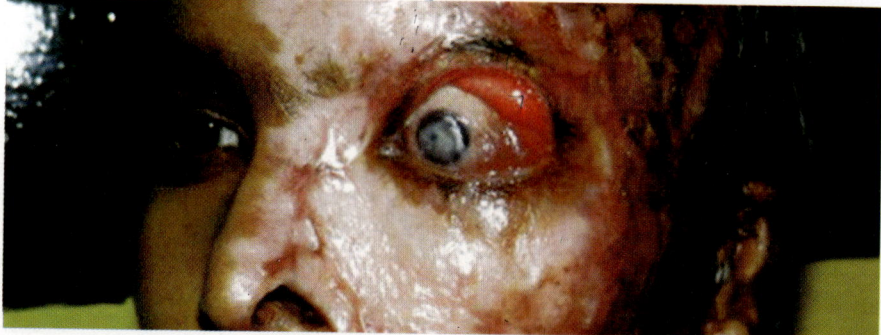

Fig. 11.1: Sulphuric acid burn injury

picture. It is helpful to remember few points:

- Weak acid penetrates freely in the living cells.
- An organic acid penetrates readily than an inorganic acid.
- Organic acid penetrates only after the surface membrane has been destroyed.
- Burn with a weak acid shows symptoms of irritation.
- Burn with a strong acid shows signs of a corrosive injury.
- As a general rule, for the acid burn, it can be said that the penetration of the ocular tissues is not marked.
- There is instantaneous cellular death. Therefore, the lesion or area of burn is sharply limited.
- The lesion is non-progressive, as further penetration of acid is prevented by the barrier offered by the precipitated proteins of the cell layer.
- The affected lesion is fixed and appears coagulated. There is no edema or disintegration of tissue affected.
- The lesion is sharply limited.
- The recovery is rapid.
- Minor and superficial burn of cornea will heal with no scar and no relapses.
- Strong acid affecting the entire cornea may result in an irrecoverable loss of the corneal tissue and so the eye.

Clinical Feature

- Irritation, lacrimation and photophobia.
- Greyish white lesions are in the epithelilal layer.
- With severe burn, the whole epithelium of the cornea is necrosed and may slough away.
- Conjunctiva is congested and may show necrosis.
- Vascularization of cornea is superficial and deep.
- Signs of iritis.
- Degenerative changes.

Management

As a general rule, the best and immediate treatment is to wash the eyes immediately without wasting a second.

Wash eyes with plenty of water. If possible the whole head can be dipped in the bucket full of water and the patient can open his eyes repeatedly in water.

In clinic, the eye physician can and should wash the eye again to be sure.

The eye must be examined with slit lamp.

Topical antibiotic eyedrops to prevent secondary infection.

Topical eye ointment twice or thrice a day depending on the extent and depth of lesion.

Some cases need steroids topically.

2. AMMONIUM HYDROXIDE BURN INJURY (NH$_4$OH—LIQUOR AMMONIA)

Young student is brought to the clinic by his teacher straight from the science college laboratory. The boy has suffered injury with ammonium hydroxide on opening the cork of the bottle. His eyes have been washed immediately with plenty of water within few seconds. He complains of lacrimation, photophobia, and intense pain.

Ocular examination show mild lid edema, marked conjunctival congestion, edema of the corneal epithelium which has been shed off at places.

Diagnosis: Chemical injury with ammonium hydroxide.

INJURY WITH AMMONIUM HYDROXIDE

Ammonia

Ammonia is available in the following forms:

- As pure ammonia (NH$_3$) in its gaseous or liquid form.
- Ammonium hydroxide, liquor ammonia (NH$_4$OH), as a solution in water. A 10% solution is used in home because of its solvent properties.
- Ammonium chloride (salt ammoniac) NH$_4$Cl.

• Ammonium carbonate (salt volatile) $(NH_4)_2CO_3$.

Thus, it can be seen that accidents are liable to occur in many circumstances, in factory or at home. At home, the accidental injury by ammonium carbonate occurs by an accidental splash or sudden forcible expulsion of gas and liquid from the domestic bottle of solution. Accidental splash on sudden forcible expulsion of gas and liquid from bottle in a laboratory occurs during the chemistry practical as it occurred in this present case.

It has been commonly used as a restorative procedure by virtue of its irritating odour, in the cases who faints due to any shock. The person is made to inhale the odour directly from the nose of bottle of ammonium hydroxide. Among all the various agents of ammonia the most common agent causing ocular injury is ammonium hydroxide.

Ammonium Hydroxide

The action of ammonium hydroxide is caustic type due to its intense alkalinity derived from the OH grouping. Its high power of solubility and penetration through the cornea makes it the most dangerous (Fig. 11.2). The usual cases seen due to ammonium hydroxide burn are from civilian population, most commonly from home or usually laboratory. As the exposure of the eye to the gas or liquid—dilute form of ammonium hydroxide is with very small quantity and there is immediate action of washing the eye therefore the damage to the eye is minimum.

Clinical Feature

• Lids are swollen.
• Intense redness of the eye due to conjunctival congestion.
• Cornea is edematous with epithelium shed off from entire cornea or at places.
• Intense lacrimation, photophobia and blepharospasm.
• Intense pain on attempt to open the eye.
• Fluorescein stain is positive.

Course

• If the injury is due to dilute ammonium hydroxide the case recovers soon within 3 to 4 days with clear cornea.
• If it is an industrial injury with ammonium and that too with concentrated ammonia and for a long-time and with no facility to wash the eye immediately within 4 to 6 seconds, then it can cause an irrecoverable damage to the cornea and the eye.
• Its high solubility and very rapid penetration makes it most dangerous.

Management

• First step is to wash the eye with water immediately.
• The eye should be washed within seconds to save the cornea from getting damaged. Wash, means pour the water in the eye with cotton swab, cloth or hanky. If possible, even dip the head in the bucket and ask the patient to open the eye in the water. It will help the patient to save his eye and sight. Force the patient to do it or do it forcibly.
• The next step is to attend the ophthalmic clinic soon.
• Meanwhile an eye ointment can be applied in the eyes.
• This treatment will be sufficient if the burn is minor and superficial.

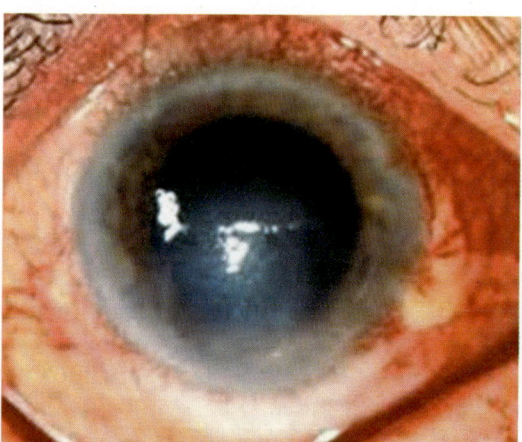

Fig. 11.2: Amonium hydroxide eye injury

- For severe case with opacification of cornea the treatment is long and difficult.

3. CALCIUM HYDROXIDE BURN INJURY (SLAKED LIME BURN INJURY)

A middle aged male enters the clinic with his left eye swollen and closed. His clothes and hands are smeared with lime. The whitewash liquid drop fell in his eyes while whitewashing the building.

Ocular examination shows intense redness of the eye more marked in the lower bulbar conjunctiva and fornix. There is chemosis. The lower part of the cornea appears denuded of epithelium. Fluorescein stain is positive in the lower part of the cornea.

Diagnosis: Burn with slaked lime (Calcium hydroxide)

Injury With Slaked Lime (Calcium hydroxide)

Calcium is widely distributed in nature and is useful for building purpose since ages. Calcium monoxide (quick lime, unslaked lime) is formed by the burning of the carbonate (limestone) in kilns. On addition of water the calcium monoxide gets converted into the calcium hydroxide (slaked lime) with generation of heat. This heat is generated first by the hygroscopic absorption of water by calcium monoxide and thereafter by chemical combination with water. The heat may increase the temperature to about 80 to 100°C. During this process of mixing a spurt of this lime is likely to get into the

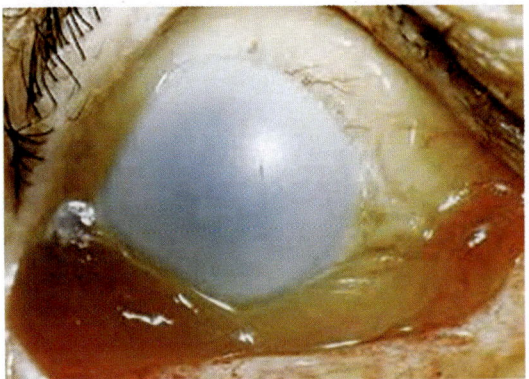

Fig. 11.3: Acute alkali burn injury showing perilimbal blenching, chemosis and corneal opacification

eyes of the worker and anyone standing nearby.

Normally, this is left overnight so that lime mixture gets cool. This is further diluted as per requirement by the worker. This diluted cool mixture of calcium hydroxide is used for whitewash. Most often the worker comes to clinic with a history of a drop falling into his eyes while whitewashing the roof. As the lime is cool and dilute and the worker washes his eyes immediately the injury caused is usually minimal. In comparison a drop of hot mixture falling into the eye while mixing the calcium monoxide with water is more dangerous. The calcium hydroxide causes trauma to the eye by the virtue of its alkalinity.

Clinical Feature

- History of splash with cool and dilute lime in the eye.
- Lids are swollen.
- Conjunctiva is congested and chemosis.
- Lower part of the cornea shows epithelial lesion.
- Fluorescein stain is positive in the area of lesion.

Course

- Slaked cool and diluted lime produces minimal injury to the eye and cornea.
- Lime in the form of powder or paste gets adherent to the ocular tissue and therefore causes more trauma.
- Calcium monoxide powder on the entry into the eye soon gets converted into the calcium hydroxide due to presence of tears and further lacrimation. At this stage it can cause more damage to the ocular tissue due to generation of heat and its being embedded into the tissues. With adherence of even a tiny particle of calcium monoxide there is intense lacrimation, photophobia and blepharospasm. If it adheres to the cornea the cornea becomes cloudy and may get opacified or necrosed depending upon the amount of calcium monoxide. If it falls into the fornix then

the conjunctiva of the fornix is intensely congested with chemosis. It may show necrosis. A case of superficial burn heals quickly. A case of deep burn may result in loss of vision and the eye.

Management

- Wash the eye with plenty of water and profusely.
- Washing of the eye should be done immediately at the site of injury.
- At the clinic eye physician should again wash taking care to wash the upper and lower fornix, so that no particle is left.
- Instillation of an antibiotic eyedrops ten times a day.
- Application of an eye ointment at bed time or thrice a day depending on each case and the extent of trauma.
- Some cases may need steroids topically in the initial stage.

General Clinical features of Chemical Burn Injury

1. In the Conjunctiva

- Congestion, itching, burning and lacrimation
- Chemosis of the conjunctiva
- Ischemia of the conjunctiva
- Necrosis of the conjunctiva
- Mucoid discharge from the conjunctiva
- Symblepharon.

2. In the Cornea

- Fine bedewing of the corneal epithelium.
- Edema of the corneal epithelium.
- Epithelium is cast-off. Fluorescein stain is positive.
- Whitish grey appearance of cornea at the site of chemical contact.
- Coagulative necrosis.
- Corrosive type of injury.
- Vascularization of the cornea the may be superficial or deep.
- Degenerative changes in the cornea.
- Complete sloughing and perforation of the cornea.

General Management

Though there is a great variation in the types of chemicals and the lesions produced by them yet the general principles of management are almost uniform.

1. Neutralisation of the Chemical Involved in Injury

Theoretically, the neutralization of the chemical which has caused the injury is the ideal and the first line of treatment. To be effective, the neutralizing agent must have following factors:

- Neutralizing agent must not damage the tissue.
- Neutralizing agent must have power of penetration as much as the chemical, causing the injury.
- Neutralizing agent must be readily available to neutralize the chemical before it produces irreversible damage to the ocular tissue.

All the above criteria cannot be satisfied except by one or two neutralizing agents. Therefore, the eye physician should think of reliable substitute to neutralize the chemical irrespective of its type, concentration and its physical state. The most reliable and easily available to anyone, anywhere, within second is the 'Water' one of the five constituents of nature. Again the nature has come to help in neutralizing the nature's chemical agent.

2. Initial Thorough Washing (Lavage) of the Eyes and Face

The first ideal treatment of chemical injury is removal of the chemical agent from the eyes and skin of the face. The rapidity without wasting even one second is very important. Thus, wash the eyes with the nearest water available and wash the affected eyes and face liberally.

- One should even ask the patient to dip his head in the bucket full of water and open the eyes repeatedly in the bucket to wash out the noxious chemical agent.

- If there is a water tap then open the tap and let the tap water flow over his head, opening the eyes in between.
- Make the patient lie down and pour water on the open eyelids with cotton swab or hanky dipped and soaked in water.
- The idea is to wash the eyes and face rapidly with plenty of water. Wash liberally. Washing will help lot to save the eyes and skin from the noxious effect of chemical agent.

Further prolong wash of the eyes

- After the initial wash the eyes can be further washed with water or saline at home or by the eye physician at his clinic.
- Irrigations of the conjunctival sac depends upon the nature and concentration of the chemical and the quantity spilled or splashed on the eyes and face.
- As a routine it is better to irrigate the eyes for at least 15 to 30 minutes at intervals. This much of time shall take care of chemicals which are slowly released from the tissues.
- If required even continuous irrigation of the conjunctival sac can be carried out with saline through the infusion set which can be so adjusted so that drops are released at the rate sufficient to keep the eye washing.

3. Removal of Particles of Chemical Agent

Examine the eye thoroughly including the fornices for any particle or particles embedded in the cornea or conjunctiva including the fornices. The particles can be removed either with irrigation and swabbing with cotton swab or by instrumentation.

Removal of chemical particles is essential as these will continue to release the active chemical agent slowly and shall continue to cause damage to the eye and tissues.

4. Fluorescein and Bengal Rose Staining

Staining shall help to know exactly the area involved. Some cases may not show stain in early period as there may be latent period for damage to epithelium especially after exposure to gases, vapours and fumes.

5. Cycloplegic

Instillation of atropine 1% eyedrops helps to alleviate the ciliary neuralgia due to association of iritis.

6. Excision of Necrotic Tissue

If there is necrosis of the conjunctival tissue then remove it early for better and early healing. The edematous and swollen corneal epithelium can be removed by a cotton—wool stick. It will help early epithelialization of the cornea.

7. Prevention of Infection

Instill antibiotic eyedrops and eye ointment as per requirement of each case to prevent superimposed secondary infection.

8. Steroids

Some cases may need steroids topically and systemically for prevention necrosis or edema.

9. Systemic Antibiotics

Course of systemic antibiotic is gratifying.

10. Acetazolamide Tablets

Some cases who are heading for glaucoma shall need course of acetazolamide for few days to keep pressure under control.

11. Prevention of Symblepharon

It can be prevented by proper application of antibiotic eye ointment. Some cases may need a mucous graft.

12. Keratoplasty

Cases with corneal opacity or necrosis of the cornea may need keratoplasty.

13. Plastic Surgery to Repair Deformity of Lids and Face

Some cases in whom there is involvement of lids and face with deformity needs plastic surgery to give them cosmetic improvement.

Alcohol Intoxication
(Ethyl Alcohol Intoxication)

Young couple enters the clinic. The wife complains that her husband shows squint when he drinks whisky of reputable brand. By the morning he appears normal to me. No other complains of any kind.

I asked her a simple question and at the same time answered it also. He must be showing the squint on getting drunk that is consuming more than his tolerance (Figs 12.1 and 12.2). Obviously the answer was, yes Doctor.

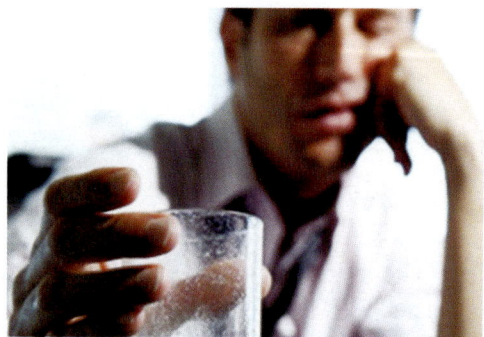

Fig. 12.1: Drinker with empty glass. Waiting to fill it up

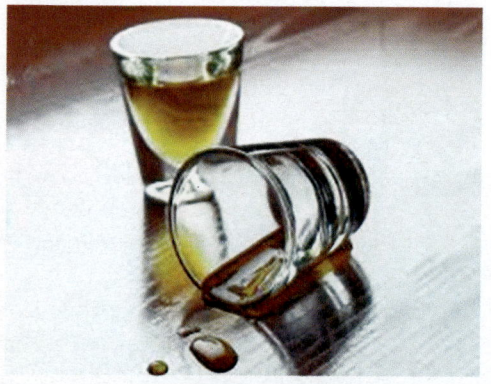

Fig. 12.2: Whisky in serving glass

Ocular examination was normal, except mild latent esophoria. Fundus appeared normal.

Visual acuity was normal.

Diagnosis: Ethyl alcohol intoxication.

ALCOHOL (ETHYL ALCOHOL) INTOXICATION

- Many organic chemicals on inhalation such as chloroform and ethyl ether produces visual disturbances preliminary to unconsciousness. The visual disturbances are due to the occurrence of diplopia and impairment of perception and judgment.
- In this class of chemicals the most important from the practical, social, family and public point of view is the consumption of ethyl alcohol by people throughout the universe irrespective of class, colour, religion or race. The ingestion of alcohol even of the reputable brand produces visual disturbances due to disturbances of higher visual functions.
- It is to be remembered and stressed that the alcohol intoxication is not a gradual process but it comes on quickly when the concentration in the blood rises to certain level which varies considerably with each individual (from 170 to 183 mg per 100 ml blood).
- The critical level is relatively constant for same individual. The effects due to concentration in the blood achieved rapidly are more potent than when the

concentration in the blood is achieved slowly. Though the intoxicating level is maintained with either rapid or slow consumption of alcohol but the time involved in a slow drink has a sobering influence.

- Therefore, the person who is addict to social drinking of alcohol must know the above facts concerning alcohol consumption. This knowledge shall keep him aware about slow drinking involving longer time period and at the same time the person should know about the amount of alcohol which he can consume without reaching critical level which will disturb the function of higher visual centres. This knowledge shall help him to keep himself safe and preserve his family also from social disrepute and accidents (Fig. 12.3).

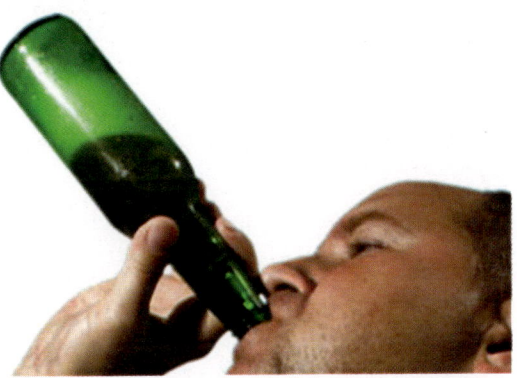

Fig. 12.3: Beer bottle of 750 ml and a drinker

CLINICAL FEATURES AND SELF-MANAGEMENT

1. Visual disturbances
2. Self-management
3. Blood alcohol testing
   a. Principle of testing
   b. binge drinking
   c. Time to sober up
   d. Hours to rid the body of alcohol
   e. Table showing progressive effects of alcohol on mind.
   f. Welcome to the frequently asked questions!

There are several visual effects which may become evident on alcohol intoxication. The manifestation of visual effects varies greatly from person to person. The most funny and important part of the alcohol intoxication is that the person denies the appearance of general depression of visual functions and rather he boost about increase in his mental and physical power. He shows indifference and lack of fear that being the visible sign of his getting intoxicated.

1. VISUAL DISTURBANCES

- Visual acuity is lowered from 5 to 20%, an appreciable amount of loss particularly in late evening or late night.
- Sensitivity to light is lowered by about 30% an appreciable loss.
- Threshold to brightness difference is increased by 50%.
- Retardation in the recovery from glare (after image) that increases considerable risk during night driving back to home.
- Disturbance in the depth perception.
- Retarded reaction time in case of breaking or blind turn on siderably dangerous while driving at night.
- General slowness in the movement of the eyes.
- Latent horizontal heterophoria always breaks down causing increase in esophoria and decrease in exophoria. Clinically, change is usually small to about 2 prism diopters yet considerable risky while driving that too after sunset and or late night.
- Decrease in the power of suppression with failed or depressed fusional ability. This results in subjective symptom of diplopia. Though the person with alcohol intoxication develops the feeling of seeing double yet he denies himself about this observation by him. The family members cannot come to know about it unless the observer can notice that he is missing to pick-up the eatables and glass also while drinking and picking eatables.
- Likely to suffer from alcoholic peripheral neuritis. If the person is habitual chronic

drinker to the extent of intoxication every day.

- If the person is also used to tobacco in any form then there are more chances for him to develop tobacco-alcohol amblyopia.
- General chronic lack of nourishment and avitaminosis (Fig. 12.4).

2. SELF-MANAGEMENT

- Abandon alcohol from menu.
- If he has to consume alcohol for social or business purpose then he must know and stay in his limit.
- Professionals are not likely to develop alcohol intoxication anytime in their life as successful persons have strong will power with creative purpose for life and family.
- In any case if professionals go out of home for social stag party then he must take care that there is non-alcoholic driver with him to drive back.
- Howsoever, small quantity he may have consumed he must not rely on his ability of judgment and reaction time.
- Successful professionals always make others drink rather than get drunk themselves.

- If at all one wishes to get drunk once in a while for fun then that professional will get drunk at home to avoid social elite to enjoy your utterly non-ethical personality and expose family and children to social taboo.
- Request and insist your sweetheart to videograph yourself intoxicated disgusting personality and show you, when you come out of your intoxication so that you can enjoy you own utterly non-presentable repelling persona. I am sure any sensible person would abandon the liquor forever, at least in social groups wherein yo are likely to be with your loved ones.

3. BLOOD ALCOHOL TESTING

Principle of Testing

Alcohol that a person drinks shows up in the breath because it gets absorbed from the mouth, throat, stomach and intestines into the bloodstream.

Alcohol: It is not digested upon absorption, nor chemically changed in the bloodstream. As the blood goes through the lungs, some of the alcohol moves across the membranes of the lung's air sacs (alveoli) into the air, because alcohol will evaporate from a

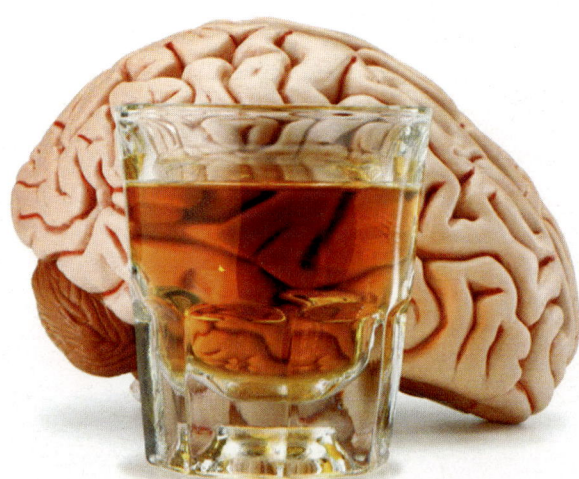

Fig 12.4: Alcohol damages all vital centres of brain leading to hellish life while alive and ending in untimely invitation to death

solution—that is, it is volatile. The concentration of the alcohol in the alveolar air is related to the concentration of the alcohol in the blood. As the alcohol in the alveolar air is exhaled, it can be detected by the breath alcohol testing device. Instead of having to draw a driver's blood to test his alcohol level, an officer can test the driver's breath on the spot and instantly know if there is a reason to arrest the driver.

Because the alcohol concentration in the breath is related to that in the blood, you can figure the blood alcohol content (BAC) by measuring alcohol on the breath. The ratio of breath alcohol to blood alcohol is 2,100:1. This means that 2,100 millilitres (ml) of alveolar air will contain the same amount of alcohol as 1 ml of blood.

For many years, the legal standard for drunkenness across the United States was 0.10, but many states have now adopted the 0.08 standard. The federal government has pushed states to lower the legal limit. The American Medical Association says that a person can become impaired when the blood alcohol level hits 0.05. If a person's BAC measures 0.08, it means that there are 0.08 gram of alcohol per 100 ml of blood (Fig. 12.5).

The body that means the liver can metabolize only a certain amount of alcohol

per hour. No matter how much or how fast alcohol is consumed, the body can only dispose of it at a rate that is generally accepted as being 1 standard drink per hour. Allowing for individual variations in weight, percent body water, percent body fat, and food intake, the amount of alcohol from one standard drink will peak, in the bloodstream, within 30 to 45 minutes.

The rapid consumption of four or five drinks in one or two hours (*see* binge drinking) overwhelms the liver with much more alcohol than it can handle. As a result blood alcohol content rapidly increases and continues to do so until drinking is stopped or decreased to a rate of less than one drink per hour. Excessively rapid drinking as frequently practiced on campus will invariably lead to dangerously high BAC levels.

Time to Sober Up

Alcohol leaves the body at conservative rate of about 0.5 oz. alcohol per hour or 0.015 percent of blood alcohol content (BAC) per hour. This is an average rate at which the liver can metabolize (burn off) alcohol. The result is that it can take many hours longer to sober up than it took to become intoxicated.

Hours to rid the body of alcohol = Peak BAC/0.015

Someone with a BAC of 0.16, or twice the legal driving limit will require over 10 hours to be completely sober and after 5 hours may still not be under the legal driving limit.

Many late night revellers never think about the time it takes to sober up. Driving or performing safety sensitive duties the morning after can put anyone at risk. If an individual's breath alcohol content is 0.20 after an evening of heavy drinking at 1:00 AM, they may not be under the legal driving limit of 0.08 BAC until approximately 9:00AM later that morning. Imagine how long it might take for the individual to be under the US Department of Transportation's BAC limit of 0.02 (Table 12.1).

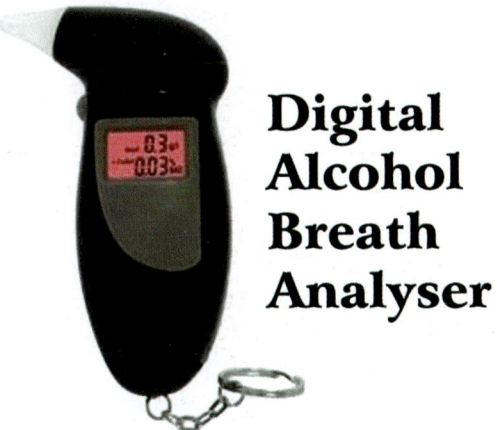

Digital Alcohol Breath Analyser

Fig. 12.5: Mini digital alcohol breath analyser to carry in pocket and measure before leaving bar. Ask for help if it has crossed the legal limit

Table 12.1: Progressive effects of alcohol on mind

BAC (% by vol.)	Behaviour	Impairment
0.001–0.029	• Average individual appears normal	• Subtle effects that can be detected with special tests
0.030–0.059	• Mild euphoria • Relaxation • Joyousness • Talkativeness • Decreased inhibition	• Concentration
0.060–0.099	• Blunted feelings • Euphoria • Disinhibition • Extroversion	• Reasoning • Depth perception • Peripheral vision • Glare recovery
0.100–0.199	• Over-expression • Boisterousness • Possibility of nausea and vomiting	• Reflexes • Reaction time • Gross motor control • Staggering • Slurred speech • Temporary erectile dysfunction
0.200–0.299	• Nausea • Vomiting • Emotional swings • Anger or sadness • Partial loss of understanding • Impaired sensations • Decreased libido • Possibility of stupor	• Severe motor impairment • Loss of consciousness • Memory blackout
0.300–0.399	• Stupor • Central nervous system depression • Loss of understanding • Lapses in and out of consciousness • Low possibility of death	• Bladder function • Breathing • Dysequilibrium • Heart rate
0.400–0.500	• Severe central nervous system depression • Coma • Possibility of death	• Breathing • Heart rate • Positional Alcohol Nystagmus
>0.50	• High-risk of poisoning • High possibility of death	• Life

FREQUENTLY ASKED QUESTIONS

Q. How does alcohol affect a person?

Ans. Alcohol affects every organ in the body. It is a central nervous system depressant that is rapidly absorbed from the stomach and small intestine into the bloodstream. Alcohol is metabolized in the liver by enzymes; however, the liver can only metabolize a small amount of alcohol at a time, leaving the excess alcohol to circulate throughout the body. The intensity of the effect of alcohol on the body is directly related to the amount consumed.

Q. What is a *standard drink*?

Ans. In different countries, health educators and researchers employ different definitions of standard unit of drink because of differences in the typical serving sizes in that country.

In the program *Alcohole-Help*, a standard drink is equal to 10 gram or 12.5 ml of pure alcohol. Generally, this amount of pure alcohol is found in:

1. 250 ml of beer
2. 100 ml of wine
3. 30 ml distilled spirits or liquor (e.g. gin, rum, vodka, or whiskey).

Q. What does moderate drinking mean?

Ans. There is no one definition of moderate drinking, but generally the term is used to describe a lower-risk pattern of drinking. Here it is defined as having no more than 1 drink per day for women and no more than 2 drinks per day for men. This definition is referring to the amount consumed on any single day and is not intended as an average over several days.

Q. What does it mean to be above the legal limit for drinking?

Ans. In India, the legal limit is 0.03 mg%.

Note: Legal limits do not define a level below which it is safe to operate a vehicle or engage in some other activity. Impairment due to alcohol use begins to occur at levels well below the legal limit.

Q. What do you mean by heavy drinking?

Ans. For men, heavy drinking is typically defined as consuming an average of more than 2 drinks per day. For women, heavy drinking is typically defined as consuming an average of more than 1 drink per day.

Q. What is binge drinking?

Ans. According to the *National Institute on Alcohol Abuse and Alcoholism (NIAAA)* binge drinking is defined as a pattern of alcohol consumption that brings the blood alcohol concentration (BAC) level to 0.08% or more. This pattern of drinking usually corresponds to 5 or more drinks on a single occasion for men or 4 or more drinks on a single occasion for women, generally within about 2 hours.

Methyl Alcohol Intoxication
(Wood Spirit Amblyopia)

Professional wood painter by profession complains of dim vision with feeling of mist in front of his eyes since last 3 months. He confessed for drinking wood spirit occasionally only when short of money to buy alcohol.

External ocular examination is normal except sluggish pupil. Ophthalmoscopy shows pale disk with attenuated retinal vessels.

Diagnosis: Methyl alcohol amblyopia

METHYL ALCOHOL AMBLYOPIA

Ethyl alcohol amblyopia manifests after prolonged ingestion of whisky.

Methyl alcohol (wood spirit) amblyopia is an acute process usually characterized by complete loss of vision and optic atrophy (Figs 13.1 and 13.2)

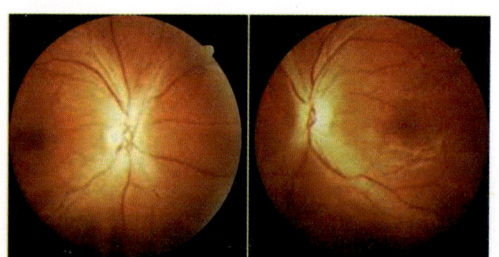

Fig. 13.1: Both eyes shows disc edema one day after drinking methanol. Usually, it ends in optic atrophy

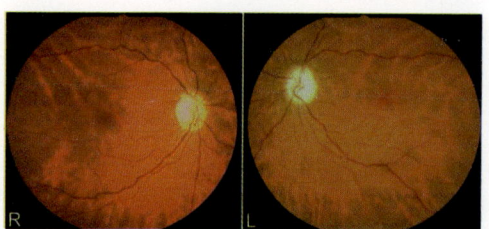

Fig. 13.2: Both eyes shows optic atrophy after few days

CLINICAL FEATURES AND MANAGEMENT

Methyl alcohol can be ingested in the following three ways:

- Most common mode is ingestion. Drinking cheap adultered or fortified beverages with methyl alcohol is the most common cause. Even tea spoonful may produce blindness and ounce is fatal resulting in death. Sometimes a habitual drinker may even drink the spirit used for the purpose of painting, etc.

- Inhalation of fumes in industry. Some cases develop addiction to inhale the methyl alcohol to get a kick.

- Absorb through skin while working with methyl alcohol industry.

The appearance of symptoms depends on the amount of consumption of wood spirit. The symptoms depend on the amount of percentage of adulteration or fortification of cheap alcohol with wood spirit by the manufacturer.

In a typical case of acute poisoning with methyl alcohol (wood spirit) the following clinical features are observed.

General Symptoms

- Headache, dizziness, nausea, and vomiting.
- Pain in abdomen.
- Prostration, delirium, convulsions, stupor, and death.
- Characteristic odour from the breath of the patient or patients is diagnostic. The odour is due to excretion of formaldehyde, the breakdown product of methyl alcohol.

is due to excretion of formaldehyde, the breakdown product of methyl alcohol.

Ocular Signs

- Pupils are dilated and fixed.
- Patient may be unable to move the eyes.
- Patient may show ptosis.
- Ophthalmoscopy shows papillitis or neuropapillitis that ends up with optic atrophy within few days.
- In less severe cases there is centro-cecal scotoma followed by gradual appearance of optic atrophy.

MANAGEMENT

- Ideal treatment in cases of acute poisoning is gastric lavage. It should be continued for 2 to 4 days, as there is evidence that the methyl alcohol in the system is continuously returning back to stomach.
- Intravenous fluids particularly sodium bicarbonate to overcome the acidosis produced by methyl alcohol.
- In severe cases peritoneal dialysis is helpful.

Glioma of Optic Nerve

Primary tumors of the optic nerve are divided into three groups:

i. *Glioma*: Ectodermal tumors of optic nerve.

ii. *Meningioma*: Mesodermal tumors of sheath of the nerve.

iii. *Melanoma*: Neuroectodermal tumors of optic nerve.

Gliomas are the most common primary tumor of the optic nerve. These are usually unilateral occurs in children and the peak incidence is 2 to 6 years of age. These grow very slowly over years and extend intracranially by direct extension along the nerve invading chiasma or through the chiasma to hypothalamus.

Glioma is a solitary tumor, non-neoplasmic and self-limiting. It may appear as a solitary spindle mass or may be spherical around the optic nerve (Fig. 14.1). Though it extends along the optic nerve it does not penetrate the dura. It presents as hypertrophic capsulated swelling without invading the surrounding structures. Usually, it extends centripetally but it may extend towards the optic disc and then to retina appearing as a solid swelling or a cyst on ophthalmoscopy.

Clinical Features and Management

Visual Disturbance

Visual loss is early and precedes the proptosis sometimes by years.

Proptosis

Proptosis is an early symptom of glioma of the optic nerve and is axial.

In later stage, the eye may be displaced downwards and outwards.

Though the proptosis is slow it may reach to endanger the cornea.

Motility of globe

In contrast to the proptosis the motility of the eye is maintained for a long-time. The eye movements are restricted once the mass has filled the orbit therefore movement is not possible due to mechanical obstruction.

Ophthalmoscopy

- In early stage the fundus is normal.
- Pressure on the globe may produce retinal striae and hypermetropic fundus.
- Effects of obstruction of circulation to the nerve may manifest as retinal hemorrhages, venous thrombosis, white exudates and star figure at the macula.

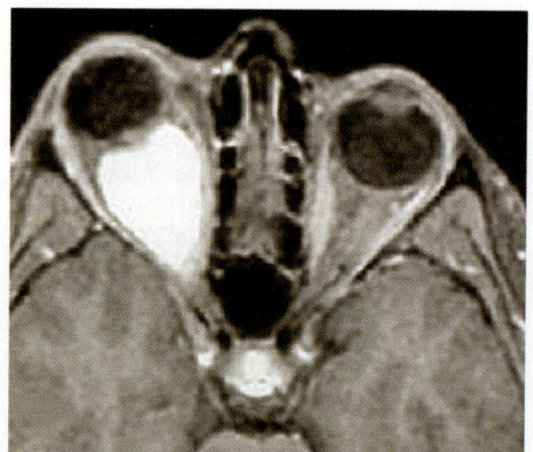

Fig. 14.1: Optic nerve glioma

- Some cases may show papilledema. Pressure on the nerve at any stage may lead to optic atrophy.

X-ray optic foramen

The spread of glioma intracranially may cause erosion or enlargement of opitc foramen.

Pathology

Macroscopically: It appears as a smooth or nodular elastic mass enclosed within the dura. On cutting the mass some cysts filled with mucinous substance are always seen. The optic nerve is compressed to one side or enclosed by the mass.

Microscopically: The picture is dominated by dense meshwork of fibrillary astrocytic processes with few nuclei.

Diagnosis

- Clinical feature of axial proptosis which is non-pulsatile, irreducible and slowly growing is one of the important diagnostic features.
- Early visual loss, presence of optic atrophy or papilledema and almost no restriction of ocular movements favour glioma of optic nerve.
- X-ray showing erosion or enlargement of optic foramen will put the diagnosis beyond doubt.
- Computerized tomography scanning will clearly demonstrate the tumor in the orbit beyond doubt.

Management

- Surgical removal if the tumor is intra-orbital. Results are gratifying.
- Treatment for restricted intracranial extension is again surgery: transfrontal approach for intracranial part and lateral orbitotomy for intraorbital part of the tumor.
- Radiation is the only treatment left for tumors which have involved chiasma.

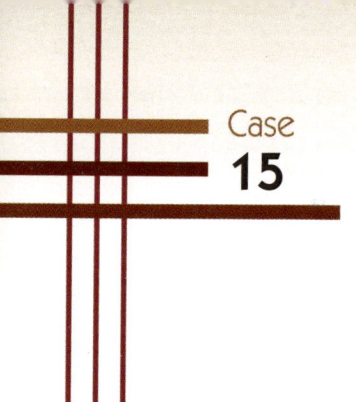
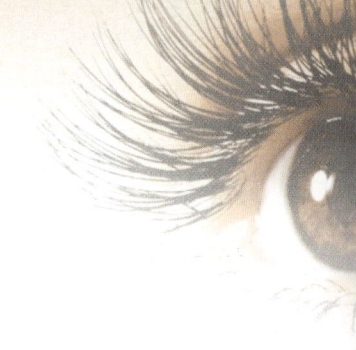

Case
15

Orbital and Paraorbital Cysts

Several types of congenital and acquired cyst can form in the orbit and periorbit region.

These usually include:

1. Dermoid cyst
2. Hydatid cyst

1. DERMOID CYST

Dermoid cysts are smooth, tense, round or hourglass shaped tumors of varying size usually of about 2 cm. The cyst is usually adherent to the underlying bone but the skin over them is freely mobile. Sometimes the underlying bone shows depression or may be absent. Then the cyst is in direct contact with the dura mater. They grow slowly in early life but grow fast at the time of puberty. These can manifest at any position along the cranial sutures.

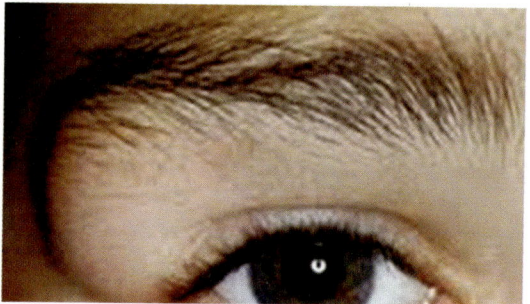

Fig. 15.1: Periorbital dermoid cyst

PERIORBITAL DERMOID CYSTS

Clinical Features and Management

These are most commonly seen at the outer and upper (frontomalar and frontoethmoid suture) or in the inner and upper (Fronto-ethmoid suture) angle of the orbit. Periorbital dermoids are known to invade the orbit secondarily in dumb-bell shape wherein intraorbital portion communicates with extraorbital portion in the temporal fossa through bony canal (Fig. 15.1).

Orbital Dermoid Cyst

Orbital dermoids are situated outside the muscle cone. These can get attached to the muscles, optic nerve or other orbital contents due to inflammation causing adhesions. Large dermoid of the orbit produces marked proptosis.

Differential Diagnosis

Cephalocele is soft, fluctuant, reducible and shows pulsation synchronous with pulse.

Histology

Dermoid cyst is lined by wall having a fibrous outer layer, connective tissue stroma with all the characteristics of skin with deposition of cholesterol crystals. A well-developed layer may be associated with papillae and contain hair follicles, sebaceous glands, sweat glands, smooth muscle, elastic fibres and deposits of calcium. The cavity of the dermoid cyst is filled with sebaceous material, hairs and desquamated epithelium.

Sometimes due to inflammatory process the cyst becomes disorganized into a soft pulpy mass.

Etiology

The occurrence of dermoid cyst is well-explained by the theory of 'dermal inclusion'.

The cyst develops from the inclusion of pouch of skin which lies dormant during fetal life.

Management

Complete surgical removal of the dermoid cyst. It is easy for periorbital dermoid cyst.

Orbital dermoids are surgically removed by lateral orbitotomy.

2. HYDATID CYST OF ORBIT (Echinococcosis)

In spite of frequency of systemic infections occurrence of hydatid cyst in the orbit is relatively rare. Hydatid cyst must be considered in the differential diagnosis of unilateral proptosis in the areas where the echinococcosis is endemic (Fig. 15.2). It affects young people without any preference for the sex or the orbit involved. In the orbit the cyst may occur at any place usually in the upper part and muscles.

Clinical Features and Management

Typical case of hydatid cyst in the orbit when fully developed gives rise to the following triad of symptoms (Fig. 15.2).

- Proptosis
- Cyst in the orbit
- Pain in the orbit.

Proptosis: Proptosis is unilateral, irreducible and non-characteristic of its direction. It is usually eccentric depending on its location. If the cyst is near the orbital margin then it may protrude as a tense, elastic swelling displacing the eye. It usually presents through the skin of the lid.

Cyst: It may fill the orbit and may be of large size. It may erode the orbital walls or may invade the cranial cavity. With its growth all the complication of extreme proptosis may occur such as keratitis, ulceration of cornea, optic neuritis, papilledema, glaucoma, and optic atrophy.

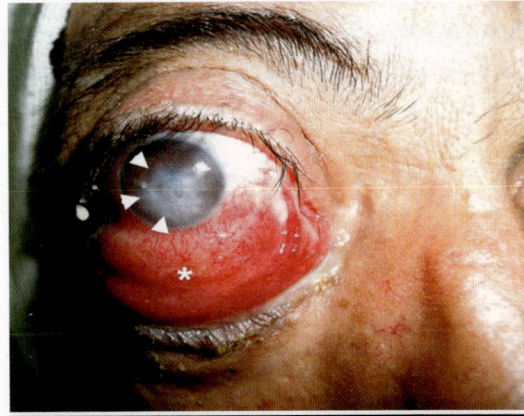
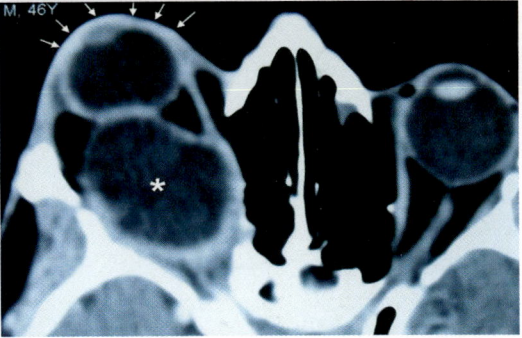

Fig. 15.2: Hydatid cyst

Pain: The pain varies in its degree from feeling of heaviness to acute neuralgia. Pain may be constant or intermittent. Any sudden exacerbation in the pain indicates either a diffusion of toxic fluid from the cyst or its local inflammation.

Diagnosis

Computerized tomography scanning shall help to locate the lesion.

Management

Surgical removal of the cyst.

In case the complete excision is not possible then cyst may be punctured and sterilized with absolute alcohol or formaline. Wash with saline and then remove the wall of the cyst.

Carcinoma of Paranasal Sinuses

1. Carcinoma of maxillary antrum, orbital apex syndrome
2. Carcinoma of frontal sinus
3. Carcinoma of ethmoid sinus
4. Carcinoma of sphenoid sinus

1. CARCINOMA OF MAXILLARY ANTRUM

The maxillary antrum is the most common site for carcinoma of paranasal sinuses invading the orbit.

The characteristic symptoms are nasal obstruction, epiphora, epistaxis and neuralgia over the area of distribution of maxillary nerve with infraorbital anesthesia.

Early diagnosis is difficult.

Presence of epiphora and associated infraorbital anesthesia in an elderly without any obvious cause must arouse suspicion.

Infraorbital anesthesia is usually the first symptom before the involvement of the bone.

The maxillary tumor is derived either from the gums or from the glands of the antral mucosa.

It tends to invade the orbital apex resulting in typical *syndrome of orbital apex* chara-cterized by ophthalmoplegia, trigeminal neuralgia and amaurosis due to involvement of the optic nerve (Fig. 16.1).

Appearance of an *orbital apex syndrome* in an elderly should arouse the suspicion of maxillary tumor. Squamous type of carcinoma has a tendency for burrowing through the tissue and bone.

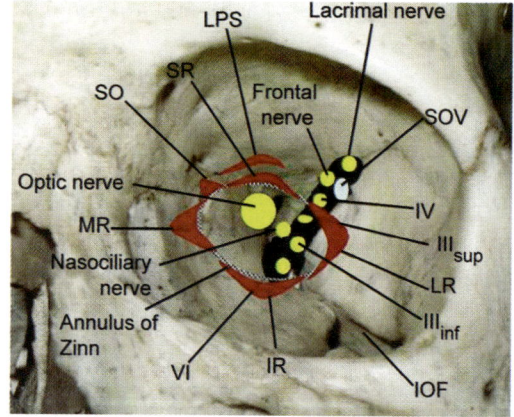

Fig. 16.1: Structures at apex of orbit

2. CARCINOMA OF FRONTAL SINUS

Carcinoma of frontal sinus is a rare phenomenon.

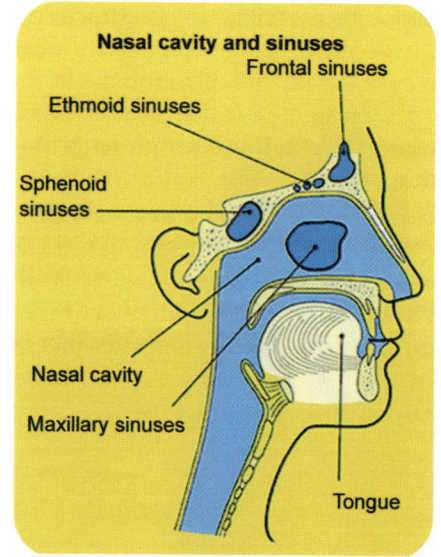

Fig. 16.2: Showing nasal cavity and sinuses

3. CARCINOMA OF ETHMOID SINUS

Carcinoma is common in ethmoid sinus. The squamous type is highly malignant. It has a tendency to invade the orbit causing proptosis and immobility of the eye.

4. CARCINOMA OF SPHENOID SINUS

Carcinoma of sphenoid sinus is relatively rare. The squamous type of carcinoma involves all the surrounding structures, including apex of the orbit. The orbital route is the most common for its spread. It causes typical orbital apex syndrome.

Treatment of Carcinoma of Paranasal Sinuses

Treatment is surgical removal. Radiotherapy can be considered either prior to surgery or post-operatively depending on stage.

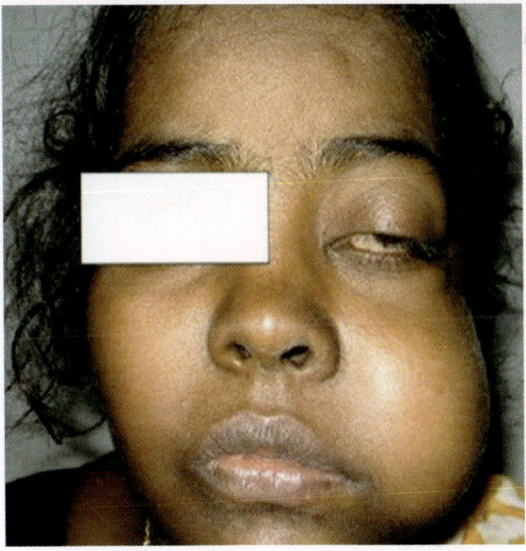

Fig. 16.3: Carcinoma maxillary sinus

Orbital Cephalocele

ORBITAL CEPHALOCELE

Cephalocele is a condition wherein a portion of contents of skull protrudes into the orbit through a defect in the wall of the orbit.

1. ANTERIOR ORBITAL CEPHALOCELE

The most common site for anterior orbital cephalocele is at the inner upper angle of the orbit or at the root of the nose (Fig. 17.1). The contents of skull protrude through the sutures between the frontal, ethmoid, lacrimal and maxillary bones. It can protrude outwards onto the face or laterally into the orbit. It may be bilateral and symmetrical.

Clinical Features and Management

It appears like a fluctuant cyst which reduces slightly under pressure. The skin of the cyst is normal but thin. Its evolution is slow. It is essential to safeguard it from trauma or pressure. In some cases cerebral symptoms such as slow pulse and convulsions might occur due to pressure on the cephalocele.

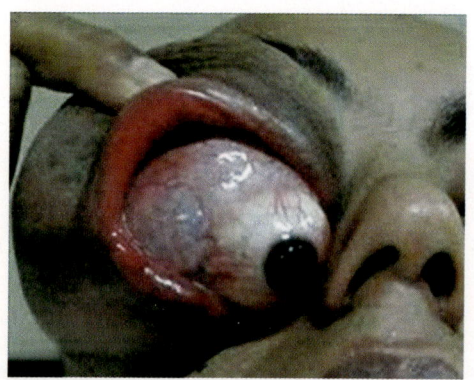

Fig. 17.1: Sphenorbital/anterior orbital encephalocele

The cyst is usually in connection with cerebral cavity by a pedicle which insinuates between cranial sutures thus creating a depression or a haitus in the bone. Presence of a hiatus is diagnostic for cephalocele. Refer case to neurosurgeon.

2. POSTERIOR ORBITAL CEPHALOCELE

Cephalocele may enter the orbit posteriorly through the optic foramen, the sphenoid fissure or through a defect in the bony orbital wall usually the suture site.

Clinical Features

It become apparent in early age or may be delayed until adult life. Its main symptom is slowly progressive proptosis with pulsation synchronous with the pulse. The proptosis is downwards and outwards with some restriction of ocular movements. This pulsating proptosis is not altered with change in the position of head or on compression of the carotids. Proptosis increases by cough, sneeze or strain. It is slightly reducible by pressure but associated with cerebral symptoms of giddiness and nausea.

Differential Diagnosis

Cephalocele is to be differentiated from dermoid. The characteristics of dermoid are largeness with well-defined margins, tenseness, no feeling of fluctuant, no reducibility, not associated with pulsation and bony defect.

Management

Consult neurosurgeon

Surgical removal by lateral orbitotomy.

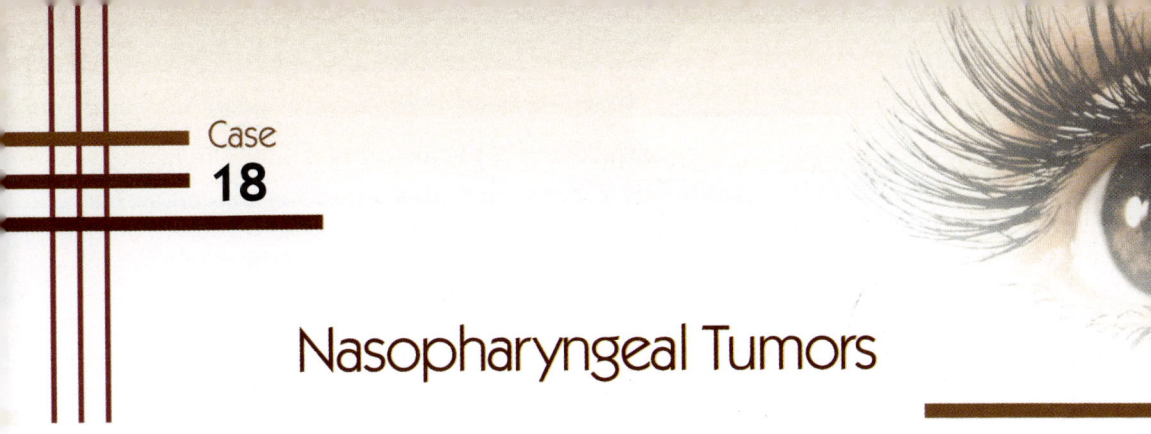

Nasopharyngeal Tumors

Nasopharynx is the upper part of the pharynx (throat) behind the nose.

Nasopharyngeal tumors cause ophthalmic disturbances due to their encroachment to the orbital apex and the base of skull. About 30 to 40% of cases present with ophthalmo-neurological symptoms.

Figure 18.1 shows three sections of nasopharynx.

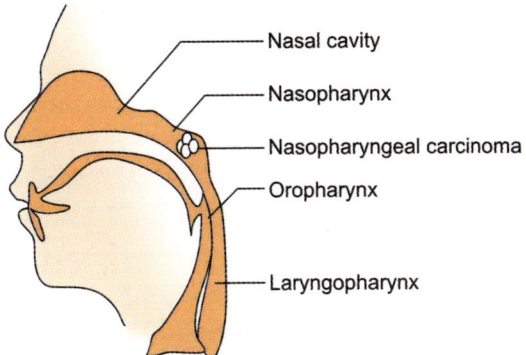

- Nasal cavity
- Nasopharynx
- Nasopharyngeal carcinoma
- Oropharynx
- Laryngopharynx

Fig. 18.1: Showing three sections of nasopharynx

A. BENIGN NASOPHARYNGEAL TUMORS

Tumors like papilloma and fibroma are rare and do not cause much complications. Adenoma and dermoids do not affect the orbit and cause no ocular complications.

1. FIBROMA

Fibroma is rare benign tumor of nasopharynx. It affects almost exclusively male adolescents, commencing at the age of puberty. The early symptoms of fibroma are: nasal obstruction, nasal discharge, epistaxis and headache. With the growth of tumor mass and involvement of other structures acute and agonising pain may occur. Other symptoms may be epiphora, diplopia, proptosis and visual loss due to compression and atrophy of the optic nerve. There may be anosmia, otalgia and deafness. Treatment is early surgical removal with or without diathermy usually through a transpalatal approach with good results. Irradiation has been considered as a method of choice due to its inaccessibility and high vascularity.

B. MALIGNANT NASOPHARYNGEAL TUMORS

1. CARCINOMA

a. Squamous Cell Carcinoma

It arises from the epithelium of the nasopharynx. It shows the epidermal characteristics of intercellular bridges and cell-nest formation.

b. Basal Cell Carcinoma

It is without cell-nests and intercellular bridges. These are invasive and destructive in their character.

c. Transitional Cell Carcinoma

It is less common. The cells are polymorphous with vesicular nuclei arranged in anastomosing cords.

d. Undifferentiated Carcinoma

There is no such a constant stable feature or pattern.

2. SARCOMA

Sarcoma of nasopharynx arises from the reticuloendothelial elements of the submucosa and is much less common than the carcinoma. These are characterized by a cytoplasmic reticulum, argentophil fibres and lymphocyte-like cells. It can occur as reticulum celled sarcoma, lymphosarcoma, fibrosarcoma and rhabdomyosarcoma.

3. PLASMOCYTOMA AND MYELOMA

Plasmocytoma arises from the plasma cells in the mucous membrane of the upper air passage. Myeloma arises from the plasma cells of the myeloid tissue of the bone and have rapid lethal course.

Clinical Features and Management

Symptoms of Nasopharyngeal Tumors

- Early and local symptoms are nasal obstruction, nasal discharge, and recurrent spontaneous epistaxis.
- Later proptosis may be the only symptom or it may be associated with ocular symptoms.
- Ocular symptoms present as 'orbital apex syndrome' or sphenoidal fissure Syndrome. There is involvement of 6th, 4th, and 3rd cranial nerves which results in irregular palsies of ocular muscles, pain

and anesthesia in the area of distribution of first division of the trigeminal nerve. Later there may be involvement of optic nerve in the form of optic neuritis or optic atrophy.

- From clinical point, any case with unexplained diplopia particularly associated with pain and anesthesia or associated with persistent otalgia and deafness without objectives signs in the ear, or with enlarged cervical lymph nodes should arouse the suspicion of a 'Retropharyngeal tumor'. Therefore, the patient should be subjected to thorough and careful nasopharyngeal examination by an expert.

Diagnosis

It is usually diagnosed late. Clinical signs and computerized tomography scanning help to arrive at diagnosis. Biopsy in some cases.

Management

It is an unrewarding problem due to its late diagnosis and marked infiltration. Surgery is not rewarding. Irradiation helps.

Dacryoadenitis

Dacryoadenitis is an inflammation of the lacrimal gland (Fig. 19.1). Inflammation may be acute or chronic. Inflammation may affect the palpebral or orbital lacrimal gland or both.

1. ACUTE DACRYOADENITIS

Etiology

- *Primary actue dacryoadenitis* may occur without any obvious etiological factor. It may follow an acute infection of the conjunctiva, upper respiratory tract and mild toxemia.

- *Secondary acute dacryoadenitis* may occur due to local or general infection.

- *Local causes* may be trauma, burn, penetrating injury and orbital cellulitis.

- *General causes* may be metastatic infection usually gonococcal and mumps.

Clinical Features and Management

a. *Acute Palpebral Dacryoadenitis*

- Patient presents with a feeling of fullness and pain in the upper and outer part of the orbit followed within few hours by inflammatory edema of the upper outer lid (Fig. 19.2).

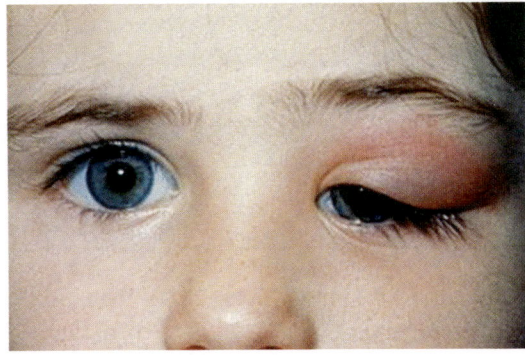

Fig. 19.2: Acute palpebral adenitis

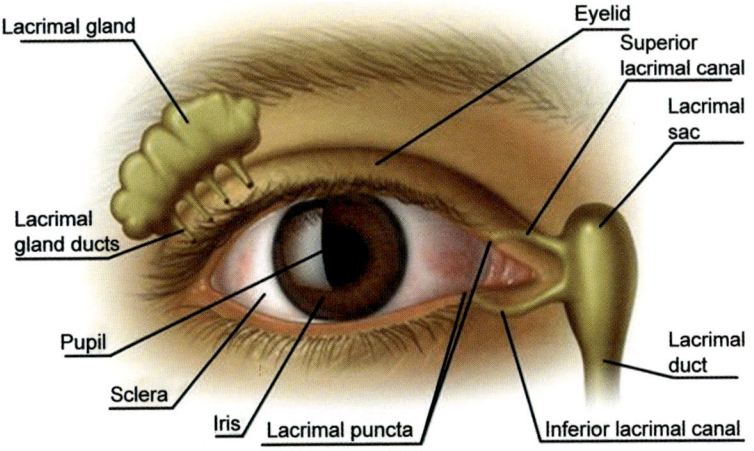

Fig. 19.1: Anatomy of lacrimal gland

Lacrimal gland
Eyelid
Superior lacrimal canal
Lacrimal sac
Lacrimal gland ducts
Pupil
Lacrimal duct
Sclera
Iris
Lacrimal puncta
Inferior lacrimal canal

- Mechanical ptosis and the upper lid margin assume typical S-shaped curve that is diagnostic for involvement of palpebral lacrimal gland.
- Edema further spreads to temple and cheek.
- Preauricular lymph nodes are enlarged and tender.
- At this stage the clinical picture resembles that of an abscess in the lid.
- Conjunctiva is chemosed and congested in the outer part.
- No disturbance in the movement of the eyeball though there is pain when the patient looks upwards and outwards and on raising the upper lid.
- General symptoms of malaise, fever and headache are present.
- It may resolve in one to two weeks or it may suppurate to discharge the pus in the conjunctival sac.

b. Acute Orbital Dacryoadenitis

As the orbital part is deeply placed all the signs and symptoms are accentuated.
- Almond shaped tender swelling under the outer orbital margin.
- Proptosis with displacement of globe downwards and inwards.
- Limitation of the movement of the eyeball in the upward and outward direction.
- Patient may complain of diplopia.
- It may resolve or suppurate to discharge pus through the skin of upper lid resulting in fistula.

Differential diagnosis

- *Acute palpebral dacryoadenitis*
  a. Abscess of lid
  b. Hordeolum
  c. Acute meibomian cyst.
- *Acute orbital dacryoadenitis*
  a. Orbital abscess
  b. Abscess from sinus
  c. Osteomyelitis of frontal bone.

Complications

- Atrophy of the lacrimal gland
- Hyposecretion of tear fluid

- Keratitis sicca
- Formation of cyst
- Formation of fistula
- Proptosis.

Management

- Early and energetic treatment with broad Spectrum antibiotics, systemically and topically can avoid suppuration and formation of fistula.
- Short course of steroids shall be helpful.
- If suppuration then evacuation is advisable rather than allow it to discharge by itself.

2. CHRONIC DACRYOADENITIS (Fig. 19.3)

Etiology

- As sequele to acute dacryoadenitis.
- Chronic local conjunctival inflammation like trachoma.
- Chronic systemic diseases such as tuberculosis, syphilis or sarcoidosis.

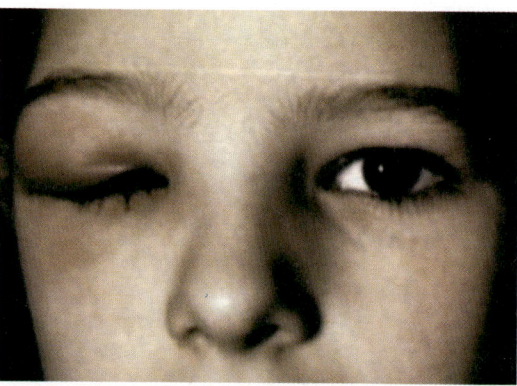

Fig. 19.3: Chronic dacryoadenitis

Clinical features

- Mobile swelling between the globe and the orbital margin.
- Globe may be pushed down and inwards.

Differential diagnosis

- Dermoid
- Sebacious cyst
- Tarsitis
- Oseteomyelitis

Management

Surgical removal is the only treatment.

Regenerative Ophthalmology: Stem Cell Treatment—A Paradigm Shift

Stem cells are the undifferentiated cells which have capacity of self renewal and differentiation. They are present in all multicellular organisms. Alexander Moximov was the Russian hematologist who postulated about stem cells.

CLINICAL FEATURES

1. Characteristics of stem cells
2. Stem cells are classified on following basis
3. Cells best suited for clinical transfers
4. Division of stem cells
5. Stem cell treatment a conceptual change: Paradigm shift
6. Indications
7. Indication for ophthalmic malady
8. Protocols for harvesting stem cells
9. Stem cell banking
10. Guidelines: Stem cell policy.

1. CHARACTERISTICS OF STEM CELLS

They have the capacity of	
Self renewal	Divide to form more stem cells
Differentiation	Convert themselves to adult somatic cells
Trans-differentiation	Stem cell of one cell line differentiates into adult cell of other cell line
Extreme mitogenic potential	Capacity to divide
Chemotaxis	Migration in response to chemical stimuli
Niche and homing	Find their comfort zone and starts living there
Chemokine activity	Cell to cell communication through protein molecules

2. CLASSIFICATION OF STEM CELL

Stem cells are classified on the following bases:

Potency	Totipotent, pluripotent, multipotent, oligopotent, unipotent
Chronology	Embryonic stem cells (ESCs), foetal stem cells (FSCs), cord blood cells (CSCs), adult stem cells (ASCs)
Characteristics	Hemopoeitic stem cells (HSCs), mesenchymal stem cells (MSCs)
Tissue of homing	Adipose tissue derived stem cells (ASCs), bone marrow stem cells (BMSCs), skin precursor cells (SPSCs), GUT
Germ line	Ectodermal, mesodermal, endodermal
Others	Very small embryonic cells (VSEL)

3. CELLS BEST SUITED FOR CLINICAL TRANSFERS

1. Multipotent
2. Adult stem cells
3. Mesenchymal stem cells
4. Adipose tissue stem cells
5. Autologus.

There are only rare indications of allogenic transfers, e.g. blood dyscrasias and cancers. Stem cells from bone marrow are rich in growth factors.

There are following known accessible sources of autologous adult stem cells in humans:

Bone marrow, which requires extraction by harvesting, that is, drilling into bone (typically the tibia, femur or iliac crest).

Adipose tissue (lipid cells), which requires extraction by liposuction.

Blood, which requires extraction through aphaeresis, wherein blood is drawn from the donor (similar to a blood donation) after pharmacological activation of bone marrow, and passed through a machine that extracts the stem cells and returns other portions of the blood to the donor.

Tooth, menstrual blood, hair follicles, skin.

4. DIVISION OF STEM CELLS (Fig. 20.1)

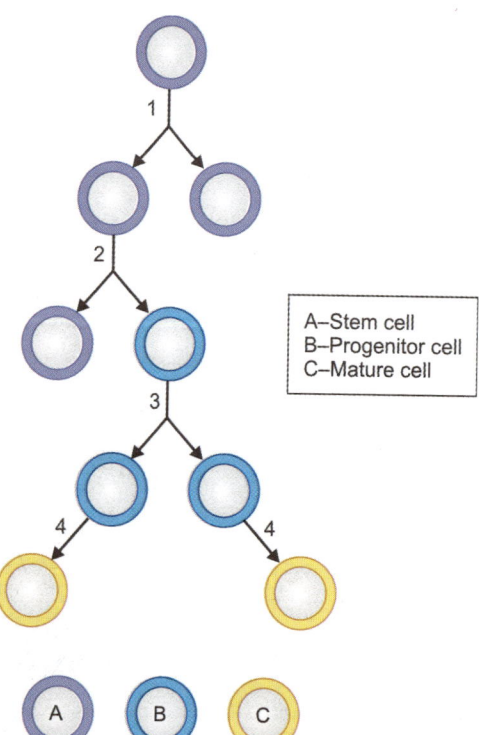

A–Stem cell
B–Progenitor cell
C–Mature cell

Fig. 20.1: Illustration showing potency of stem cells at various stages of development

5. STEM CELL TREATMENT—A CONCEPTUAL CHANGE: PARADIGM SHIFT

Stem cell treatment is a conceptual change in the treatment of those diseases where the outcome of disease is poor and cannot be treated by existing modalities of treatment. For most of the diseases like traumatic paraplegia, motor neurone disease, cerebral palsy, optic atrophy, alopecia, cirrhosis liver, age related macular degenerations, retinitis pigmentosa, diabetes mellitus type 1 patient leads a vegetative life and considered to be a burden in the family and society.

Traumatic paraplegia	20 lakhs patients in India
Cerebral palsy	25 lakh patients in India
Neurological disorders	68 lakh people die every year worldwide
Optic atrophy	12 lakhs patients in India

Data mentioned above is quite alarming. In a third world country like India this is a potential health problem which requires treatment and rehabilitation

Research on **stem cells** continues to advance knowledge about how an organism develops from a single cell and how healthy cells replace damaged cells in adult organisms (Fig. 20.2). Stem cell research is one of the most fascinating areas of contemporary biology, but, as with many expanding fields of scientific inquiry, research on stem cells raises scientific questions as rapidly as it generates new discoveries.

6. INDICATIONS

Stem cells transplantation is done for diseases of all system like musculoskeltal system, nervous system, cardiovascular system, respiratory system, endocrine system, immune system, genitorurinary system. Stem cells are used for antiaging, cosmetic purpose, blood dyscrasias and cancers also.

7. INDICATION FOR OPHTHALMIC MALADY

1. Optic atrophy
2. Age related macular degeneration
3. Stargards disease*, Bests disease*

*We have treated Stargards macular dystrophy by giving 1 ml intravitreal injection BE and the vision improved from hand movement BE to 6/60 BE and Bests disease by giving 1 ml intravitreal injection in 1 eye only and the vision improved from 6/60 to 6/12. Both the patients improved after the treatment.

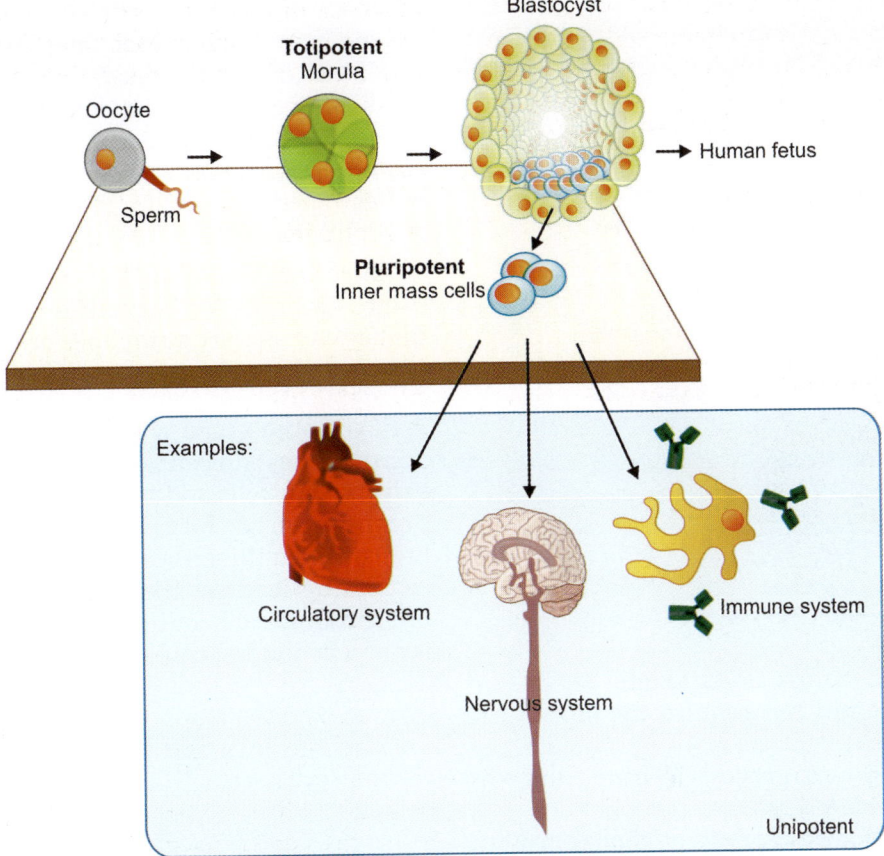

Fig. 20.2: Concept of stem cell treatment

4. Retinitis pigmentosa
5. Corneal opacities
6. Bullous keratopathy

The ideal dose of stem cells for ophthalmological indication is 10 million each eye. Stem cells can be given by retrobulbar injection, intravitreal injection, in retina by creating artificial retinal detachment, intrathecally (lumbar puncture) and IV.

8. PROTOCOLS FOR HARVESTING STEM CELLS

1. Bone marrow
2. Adipose tissue

Bone marrow: Through specialized bone marrow aspiration cannula, bone marrow is harvested from iliac crest then isolated, concentrated, and stabilized. The concentrated extract is then injected (CD 34 and 45).

Adipose tissue: Liquefying fluid (tumescent) is injected into fat area from where stem cells are to be harvested. Than this tissue is subjected to enzyme digestion by lecithin or collagenase and than centrifuged. Concentrate from this tissue contain large quantity of mesenchymal stem cells (CD 73, 90 and 105).

9. STEM CELL BANKING (Fig. 20.3)

Stem cells for banking are procured either from cord blood, cord tissue or tooth germ. This concept is dying out because of following reasons:

- Cells are not fresh.
- Life is 21 years.
- Cells cannot be cultured, only few million cells, ideal dose is 1 million/kg.
- Only 50–60 ml blood is stored.
- Leave out cord tissue which is rich source of mesenchymal cells.

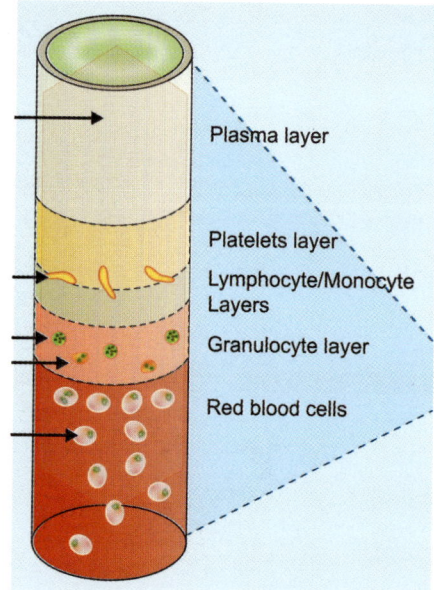

Fig. 20.3: Stem cell banking

Plasma layer

Platelets layer

Lymphocyte/Monocyte Layers

Granulocyte layer

Red blood cells

- Cost of storage is very high.
- One might not require the stored cell (20000:1).
- When we can harvest cell from adult why to use stored cells.
- They might go karyotype change or aging in artificial media.
- FDA condemns it.

10. GUIDELINES: STEM CELL POLICY

Clinical use of stem cells is not permitted until the efficacy and safety of the procedure is established; origin, safety and composition of the product is adequately defined and labelled; and conditions for storage and use are given in detail. Guide lines are framed by ICMR, CBT, and under drug and cosmetic act. ICMR had laid the guidelines regarding the research into stem cell.

- Permissible area
- Restricted area
- Prohibited area

There are ethical issues involved with the use of embryos for harvesting stem cells, that's why stricter guidelines are laid.

11. STEM CELLS FUTURISTIC SCIENCE

A day would come when doctors can do organogenesis of entire eyeball with the help of stem cells and transplant it, though presently we can form a few parts with the help of three dimensional grafting of stem cells using scaffold. Stem cells are nothing but the craftsman crafting the eyeball, this is not a fiction but true analysis (Fig. 20.4).

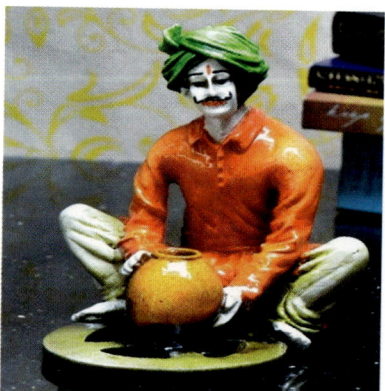

Fig. 20.4: Craftsman crafting pot

Part 2

Specific Common Symptomatic Cases

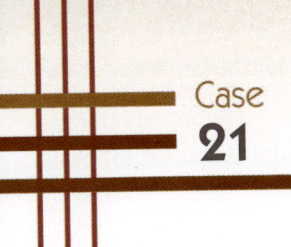

Crab Louse
Infestation of Lashes

Young lady along with her son about 4 years in age enters the clinic with anxiety and points towards the lashes of her son's eyes. The child is rubbing the eyes constantly. She has noticed peculiar knots almost all over the upper lashes. Ocular examination shows dark minute nits on the lashes.

Diagnosis: Crab louse infestation of lashes.

CRAB LOUSE INFESTATION OF LASHES

- Crab louse is normally an infestation of pubic hairs around the genital organs.
- Crab louse infestation of eye lashes is more common than the infestation of brows and scalp hairs (Fig. 21.1).
- Infestation with crab louse of the lashes and eyebrows has been recorded from very early times (Fig. 21.2).
- Though it seems unbelievable I have encountered cases infested with crab

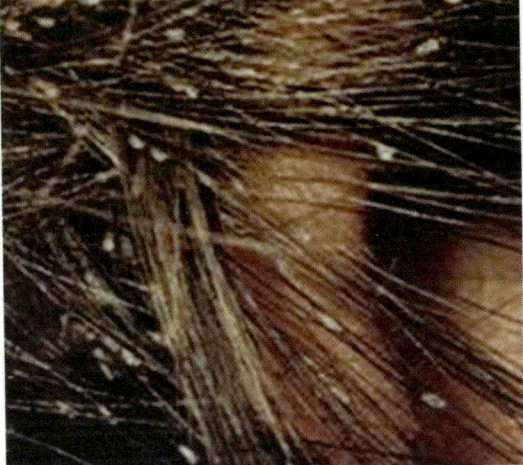

Fig. 21.2: Eggs or nits of crab lice infestation of scalp hairs

louse in the children from families of high social status with clean, well-ventilated hygienic living conditions.
- When the parents particularly mother is told about the crab louse infestation she resists to believe (Fig. 21.3).

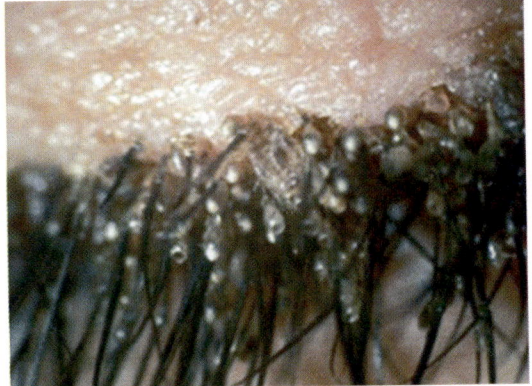

Fig. 21.1: Eggs or nits of crab lice at the root of eyelashes

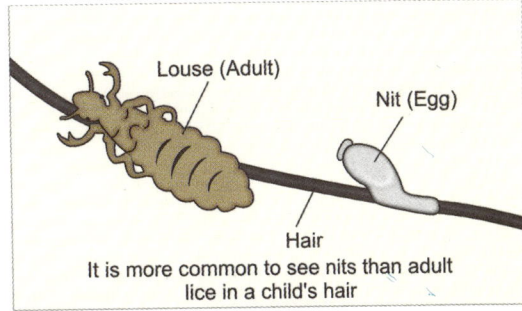

Louse (Adult)

Nit (Egg)

Hair

It is more common to see nits than adult lice in a child's hair

Fig. 21.3: Shows egg and lice. It is more common to see nits than adult lice in kids

- On enquiry and clinical examination the maid or mistress who looks after the child is found to be infested with the crab louse of pubic and scalp hairs.
- The crab louse reaches eye lashes by the transmission of crab louse from pubic hairs through hand or fomite.
- Involvement of lashes, brows and scalp hairs without infestation of pubic hairs is rare.
- The infestation is commonly seen in children from slums due to prevalence of unhygienic living conditions.

Clinical Features

Crab Louse Infestation of Lashes and Eyebrows

- Large number of crab louse can be seen gripping on to the roots of the eyelashes or eyebrows with their claws.
- The ova are deposited on the eyelashes. These remain adhering to the lashes and appear as nits of dark colour almost involving all the lashes.
- The crab louse is not visible but the tell-tale nits on the lashes are easily and readily visible. One cannot miss this nit of ova adhering to lashes along their length.
- Patient feels itching and therefore not only rubs the eyes rather scratches the lid margin with his finger nail. This scratching by fingernail leads to inflammation of lid margin.

Scalp Hair Louse Infestation

Head louse infestation may be seen on the lids involving the lashes along with the infestation of the scalp.

Head louse bite to suck the blood from the lid margin. This leads to itching, scratching and secondary infection of the lid margin. This results in chronic blepharitis. The head louse and ova are attached to the hairs about 3 mm from the skin.

Management

To remove crab louse from scalp hair, eye-lashes and brows along with nits is very difficult process.

So, trim the eyelashes and browlashes up to roots. Pick-up louses by forceps under operating microscope/magnifying loupe.

Delouse the source to prevent re-infestation.

Topical antibiotic eyedrops four times and ointment at bed time for 2 weeks.

Prevention is better than cure. Be awake to keep the maid live with cleanliness.

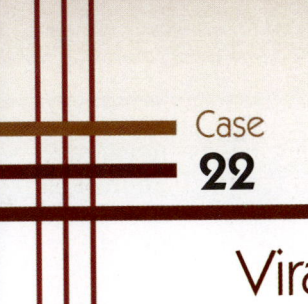

Viral Inflammation (Vesicles) of Lids

Patient attends the clinic with small vesicles on the lids with complains of mild discomfort in the eyes, lacrimation, scanty discharge coupled with history of fever preceding the appearance of vesicles.

Ocular examination shows a few vesicles on the lids. There is mild conjunctival congestion.

Diagnosis: Viral inflammation (vesicles) of lids.

VIRAL INFLAMMATION (VESICLES) OF LIDS

- Viral infections of the lids are becoming more and more common.
- Some of these produce mild symptoms and are difficult to diagnose and treat.
- Some of these produce acute signs and symptoms and need early and energetic treatment to avoid complications.
- Viral infections which assume an acute exanthematous form also involve the eyelids in the same way as the rest of the skin.
- Thus, it shall be of interest that we discuss here the viral infections of lids in detail.

CLINICAL FEATURES AND MANAGEMENT

1. Vaccinia
2. Herpes simplex
3. Herpes zoster
4. Warts
5. Molluscum contagiosum
6. Measles
7. Chickenpox

1. VACCINIA

Infection of lids with vaccinia virus is not very rare. It is usually an accidental infection of lids with vaccinia virus.

Clinically, it occurs in two forms:
 i. Vaccinial pustule
 ii. Vaccinial blepharitis

Vaccinial Pustule

Vaccinial pustule occurs at the site of inoculation on the outer surface of the lids. After an incubation period of three days one can see a few coalescing vesicles within the zone of erythema at the site of inoculation. The lids are intensely swollen with pre- and post-auricular lymphadenopathy. By 9th day the patient develops general symptoms of fever and malaise. Lid vesicles gradually become purulent and show crusting after 12th day. The curst falls off and an ulcer is formed surrounded by granulations and the floor covered with thick grey necrotic material. This necrotic material eventually falls off to leave red pitted scar. Healing is very good.

If the patient has already been vaccinated earlier then the lesion is very mild assuming the form of an itchy papule which develops in a shallow pustule and a shallow ulcer. The ulcer heals leaving a shallow red pitted scar. Though the lid margin is not involved yet corneal complication in the form of disciform keratitis may develop.

Vaccinial Blepharitis

Vaccinial blepharitis affects the lid margins. The ulcer so formed may spread over the palpebral conjunctiva. The ulcer presents a thick dirty grey membrane. There is no scab formation. The infection may spread to lid surface and may cover large areas. Healing occurs in about 10 days with thickened lid or distortion of lid margin. Symblepharon and disciform keratitis may occur as complications.

Treatment

- Inject vaccinal γ-globulin intramuscularly 1500 mg.
- Topical instillation of γ-globulin—250 mg in distilled water, as eyedrops.
- Acyclovir ointment—5 times a day. A course of oral tetracycline along with vitamins, minerals and nourishing diet.

2. HERPES SIMPLEX (Fig. 22.1)

- Infection may be acquired at birth from vulva of the mother. Usually, the child is protected for the first six months of his life by circulating maternal antibodies. The infant is prone to virus inoculation most frequently due to kiss in the region of lids or cheeks offered by relatives, friends and visitors as customary ritual.
- If the infant escapes inoculation then the child is again at risk of inoculation at adolescence by kiss from his or her friends.

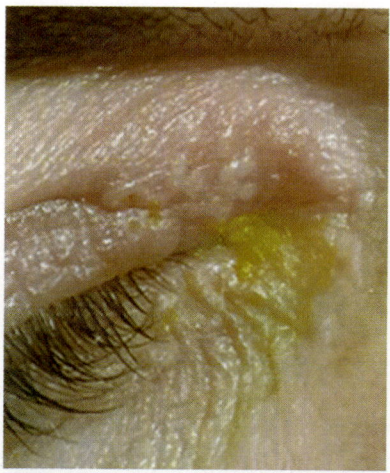

Fig. 22.1: Vesicle of herpes simplex

- Once the inoculation has been acquired the virus remains latent. It manifests by some extraneous factors usually an attack of coryza or fever involving upper respiratory tract or body complex. Psychological factor has been blamed.

Clinically

Vesicles appear in crop of pinhead size on the lids, lips or both. To begin with the vesicles are filled with clear yellow fluid. In few days the vesicles dry to form a yellow-brown crust which falls off in about seven days.

An acute follicular conjunctivitis and keratitis may occur as complication.

Treatment

- Treat by topical application of acyclovir.
- Other drugs are cytarabine (cystosine arabinoside) and vidarabine.
- Systemic tetracycline is helpful in preventing secondary infection.

3. HERPES ZOSTER

Herpes zoster affects older person in whom the dorsal root ganglion of the cord or the extramedullary ganglion of the cranial nerves both sensory and motor get involved and manifest as vesicles in the area of distribution of the nerve.

Herpes zoster is of importance to an ophthalmologist when the gasserian ganglion is involved mainly affecting the first division but two or all the three divisions of faith cranial nerve may be involved.

Clinically

Onset is sudden with fever and neuralgic pain over the distribution of first division of fifth cranial nerve. Soon in 3 to 4 days there is blushing of the skin followed by marked edema, swollen lids and vesicles. To begin with the vesicles are filled with clear fluid which soon becomes turbid and yellow. These vesicles burst forming scabs which fall off leaving deep pitted scars.

Neuralgic pain along the severe tenderness of the skin may persist for months or years.

It is aggravated by slightest contact even by drought of air or mild touch with hand or comb. The affected area of skin shows diminished sensitivity and numbness and if associated with neuralgic pain then it is known as a condition of *anesthesia dolorosa*.

Ocular Complications

Zoster may be accompanied or followed by complications particularly if the naso-ciliary branch of first division of fifth cranial nerve has been involved:

- Conjunctivitis
- Keratitis
- Uveitis
- Retinitis
- Optic neuritis
- Ocular palsies

It is essential that a careful watch should be kept on the eye to diagnose and treat these complications early.

Treatment

- Topical application of acyclovir ointments, anesthetic gel and poison.
- Systemic steroids in high-dose give favourable results.
- Systemic analgesics provide relief from pain.

4. WARTS

Warts are small autoinoculable epidermal and papillary masses caused by a filterable virus.

Clinically

Wart appears as tiny grey irregular, horny, single or multiple, discrete or coalescing, flat or filiform growths on the skin of lids. These occur due to infection being carried to lids from elsewhere. Warts produce no symptoms except cosmetic embarrassment. If the warts appear at the lid margin between the eyelashes then it is followed by follicular conjunctivitis or keratitis.

Treatment

- Surgical removal of warts. Excise or scrap and touch the base of warts with poison or silver nitrate.

- With excision of warts all the symptoms of conjunctivitis or keratitis disappear in short-time.

5. MOLLUSCUM CONTAGIOSUM

Molluscum contagiosum is characterized by small globular umblicated vesicles on the skin of lids and at the lid margin. It is mildly contagious disease caused by filterable virus (Fig. 22.2).

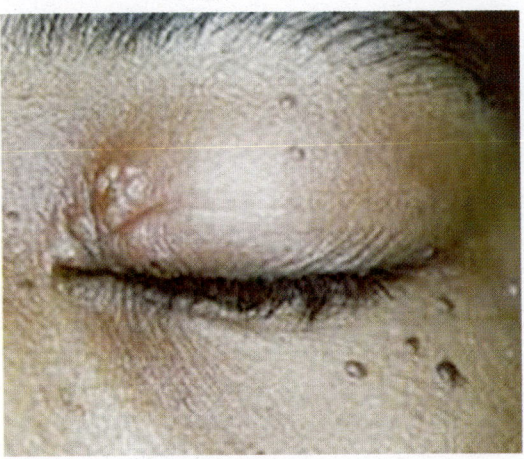

Fig. 22.2: Vesicles of molluscum contagiosum

Clinically

Vesicles appear as small pimples, discrete or multiple spread over the lids. Vesicles are typically globular with broad base and a flat umbilicated top with a small tiny dark spot in the centre. To begin with these globular vesicles are firm and solid but gradually soften. On squeezing they exude waxy like material resembling sebum. Sometimes these vesicles burst and disappear spontaneously. Usually, persist for months or years. If located at the lid margin then these vesicles lead to chronic follicular conjunctivitis and superficial punctate keratisis. These ocular complications are probably due to allergy to toxins of the virus. The virus does not invade the conjunctiva or cornea. The follicular conjunctivitis is mistaken for trachoma especially due to presence of associated pannus.

Treatment

- Surgically incise the globular vesicles by sharp pointed knife and squeeze out the contents.
- Swab the cavity with carbolic acid or tincture of iodine to prevent recurrence.
- Results are gratifying.

6. MEASLES

Measle is general viral infections. These may involve the eyelids also.

- These may be associated with acute or chronic conjunctivitis.
- There is always some lid edema associated with these as a part of general infection.

- These cases should be managed properly in isolation to prevent infection to other members of the family especially children. Needs supportive general line of treatment.

7. CHICKENPOX

Chickenpox is characterized by cutaneous rash that is usually vesicular but may become pustular. The vesicles develop into an excavated ulcer with marked edema of the lids. It is self-limiting and lesion regresses leaving pitted scar. Treat by bland lotions and supportive needs.

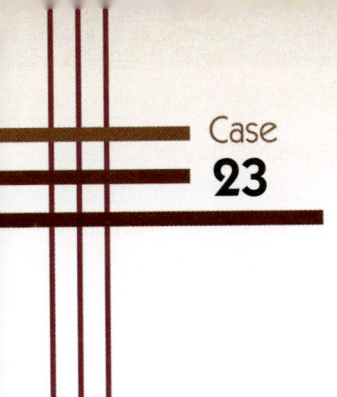

Lid Edema

Patient attends the ophthalmic clinic with edema of the upper lid with mild discomfort. He saw the edema of the lid in the morning and has come for consultation within hours.

Ocular examination shows mild lid edema of the upper right lid. There is no pain or tenderness.

Diagnosis: A case of lid edema.

LID EDEMA

Edema of lids is a symptom complex of many ocular and systemic pathological conditions characterized by increased permeability of the lid capillaries with laxity, distensibility and retaintivity of the subcutaneous connective tissue of the lid (Fig. 23.1). There is permeation of fluid due to increased capillary permeability and the lid's connective tissue has enough laxity to withhold the permeated fluid. The fluid collected in the lids is prevented to extend

to forehead and cheek due to the strong facial attachments at the brow and naso-jugal and malar folds.

In the inflammatory lid edema the skin is hot and red in appearance.

When the lid edema is on the increase then the skin of the lid appears smooth and tense. When the lid edema is subsiding then there appears fine wrinkling over the skin of lids—a sign of resolution.

Lid edema appears even from a trivial cause. It may be acute and massive to close the eye mechanically. Therefore, it is frightening to the patient and that forces the patient to attend the ophthalmic outpatient or ophthalmologist. It is very important to inspect the palpate the lid thoroughly so as not to miss a small, almost undetectable stye, chalazion or sting from insect.

Careful history helps in diagnosis.

ETIOLOGICAL FACTORS

1. *Inflammation of the lids*:
    – Hordeolum externum (stye)
    – Hordeolum internum (acute meibomitis)
    – Cellulitis and abscess of the lids
    – Sting of insect
2. *Inflammation of the orbital tissue*:
    – Orbital cellulitis
    – Tenonitis
    – Periostitis
    – Myositis
    – Orbital thrombophlebitis
3. *Intracranial inflammation*:
    – Cavernous sinus syndrome

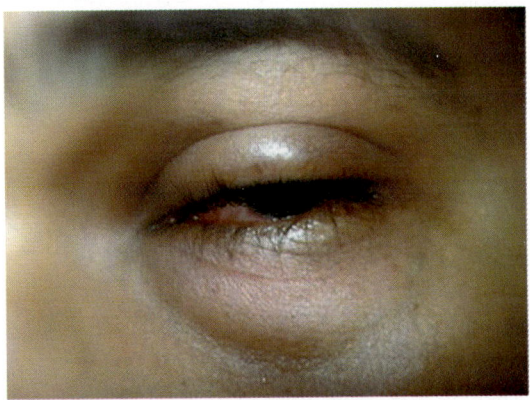

Fig. 23.1: Lid edema

4. *Paranasal sinus inflammation*
5. *Inflammation in the scalp*:
   – Dandruff of scalp hairs
   – Eczematous dermatitis

NON-INFLAMMATORY LID EDEMA

1. Lymphodema
2. Allergic and vascular edema:
   – Urticaria
   – Angioneurotic

CLINICAL EXAMINATION

Inspection

Inspect the lid in good day light, spot torch or even with slit-lamp. In acute and massive edema of lid that overhangs the lower lid then inspect the eye with lid retractor.
- Look for the extent of edema.
- Is there any specific margin or not?
- Skin is tense and smooth in edema of lids.
- Any pus point, vesicles or sting of insect over the edematous lid.

Palpation

- Palpate the lids softly and gently with the pulp of the index finger or thumb so as not to excite any pain.
- Palpation is essential as a small cyst of meibomian gland may be missed on inspection.
- Palpation also gives information about any specific point of pain which may be the site of undetectable stye or sting of insect.

Conjunctiva

Examination of the conjunctiva is very essential in all the cases especially wherein the lid edema is causing closure of lids.

Eversion of Lid

- Eversion of lids may help you to arrive at the diagnosis.
- Double eversion of lid may be required in some cases wherein it is essential to examine the fornices.

CLINICAL FEATURES AND MANAGEMENT

1. Lymphodema
2. Allergic and vascular edema
3. Eczematous dermatitis
4. Cellulitis and abscess of lids.
5. Hordeolum externum (stye)
6. Hordeolum internum (acute meibomitis)

1. LYMPHEDEMA

Lymphedema is due to defect in lymphatic drainage which when becomes chronic leads to development of firm, non-pitting swelling of the lid associated with epidermal thickening and accumulatin of lymphocytes and plasma cells in the sub-epidermal tissue. It is known as 'solid edema'. Solid edema of the lid is common in generalized hypertrophy of cutaneous and subcutaneous tissue of the lids following chronic or recurrent edema. Most common cause is *chronic eczema or recurrent erysipelas*.

Most common cause for secondary lymphodema is recurrent erysipelas. The other common cause is granulomatous tumor of orbit in which there are no inflammatory signs but the lid shows edema in which fingers can sink but not pitted. The lid is large and heavy. This is most probably due to blockage of lymphatic drainage.

Differential diagnosis in a case of solid edema of lid includes fibroma, lipoma, neurofibroma and leukemic infiltration. Solid edema may eventually lead to permanent hypertrophy or elephantiasis.

Elephantiasis is due to stagnation of an extracellular fluid rich in proteins which leads to cellular infiltration and fibrosis. Elephantiasis can be primary or secondary. Elephantiasis due to filarial infestation is well-known entity attacking the lower extremities.

2. ALLERGIC AND VASCULAR EDEMA

Allergic edema mainly affects the dermis and subcutaneous tissue preferentially. Lid appears puffy. Usually, the patients are of nervous nature. Many of these are having chronic colitis. Any stimulation can cause this type of edema.

Urticaria

Urticaria is an acute edema characterized by appearance of weals of edema due to transudation occurring in the dermis and subcutaneous tissue of the lid. It is in response to the local release of histamine-like substances from the mast cells of the skin. Lid edema may be more generalized rather than having sharp edge weals. The phenomenon is hypersensitive reaction of anaphylactic type.

Angioneurotic Edema

It is a chronic condition of vasomotor origin affecting mainly the subcutaneous tissue. The lesions are tense, round and non-pitting. The overlying skin is normal. There is no itching over the spot of edema. It can occur due to allergic, endocrine or toxic disturbances. It is a hypersensitive reaction of anaphylactic type. Both types of edema allergic and angioneurotic may be seen in the same patient.

3. ECZEMATOUS DERMATITIS

Eczematous dermatitis is inflammatory reaction characterized by varied clinical features: erythema, papules, vesicles, and patches which may be scaly, weeping or crusted, associated with a sensation of burning and itching.

Eczematous dermatitis of lid is usually accompanied by blepharitis, conjunctivitis or even keratitis. Etiologically, it can occur due to a primary irritant or as an allergic dermatitis.

Eczematous dermatitis can be of acute, subacute or chronic type. Most often it is of chronic type with recurrences. The skin of lid forms a common site for an eczematous dermatitis because of its delicate structure and exposure to atmosphere.

Management involves the treatment of eczema of surrounding area especially of scalp and prevention of secondary infection.

Pay attention to the mental health of patient.

Steroids, local and systemic, have given good response.

Treat the causative factor if found.

4. CELLULITIS AND ABSCESS OF THE LIDS

Cellulitis and abscess formation in the lids occur due to purulent inflammation.

Etiology

1. *Exogenous*: Any trauma in form of erosion, rupture or tear of the lid can be responsible for introduction of infection. A trauma which leads to formation of a hematoma is likely to become an abscess if not taken care of with proper antibiotics.
2. *Metastatic cellulitis*: It can occur due to metastatic infection through the blood stream as in pyemia.
3. *From neighbouring inflammation*: Cellulitis of lids can occur following infection of lid such as stye, furuncle, hordeolum, gonococcal conjunctivitis, orbital periostitis, dacryocystisis and sinusitis.

Clinical Features

- In early stage there is brawny infiltration with swelling of the lid. The skin over the lid is red, tense and hot to feel.
- Due to intense swelling of the lid it is usually not possible to localize the spot of infection or trauma.
- The regional lymph nodes preauricular and mandibular are enlarged and tender.
- Patient usually presents with general symptoms of fever and malaise.
- Later there is abscess formation which may breakthrough the skin to discharge or the overlying skin shows sloughing and necrosis.

Treatment

- Systemic antibiotics, preferably intravenous.
- Application of moist heat.
- Incision and drainage in cases with pus point.
- Surgical dressing in cases with sloughing and necrosis.

5. HORDEOLUM EXTERNUM (STYE)

Hordeolum externum is an acute suppurative infection of the ciliary follicle involving the associated gland of Zeis. The most common causative organism is *Staphylococcus*.

Etiology

It arises as a pure infection of ciliary follicle and can be associated with debility and diabetes. A focal infection of the upper respiratory tract favours its occurrence. It can also arise as complication of acne vulgaris.

Clinical Features

The inflammation of the ciliary follicle usually presents with lid edema of the upper or lower lid or both the lids (Fig. 23.2).

The edema may be circumscribed or may be widespread involving the whole lid more nearer the lid border.

Soon there is appearance of red indurated swollen area on the lid margin. This indurated area soon shows a yellow point of pus on the lid margin around the root of an eyelash.

In few days the skin gives way and pus is discharged leaving a central slough area. The swelling subsides and the wound heals with cicatrization which may result in an isolated trichiasis.

It may appear in crop or one after another over a long period or there may be multiple styes all in different stage of evolution.

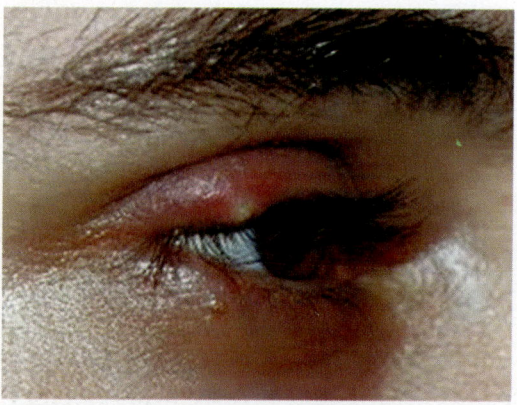

Fig. 23.2: Stye upper lid

Patient comes with marked edema of lid with pain and tenderness at localized spot on the lid margin. In early stage the pain is sharp and cutting type. With formation of pus the pain becomes dull and throbbing. The pain subsides with discharge of pus.

Complications

- Cellulitis of the lid with or without abscess formation
- Orbital thrombophlebitis
- Orbital cellulitis
- Cavernous sinus thrombophlebitis
- Meningitis
- Staphylococcal septicemia.

Treatment

- Systemic antibiotics
- Topical instillation of antibiotic eyedrops and ointment
- Hot fomentation twice a day until the pus point is seen
- Do not open the stye until there is a pus point
- If there is pus point then incision is the best treatment
- Analgesics to provide relief from pain.

6. HORDEOLUM INTERNUM (ACUTE MEIBOMITIS)
Etiology

Hordeolum internum is acute suppurative infection of the meibomian gland. The most common causative organism is *Staphylococcus*.

Clinical Features

- In its early stage it presents with pain and inflammatory edema of the upper lid.
- There is localized spot of tenderness which indicates the site of lesion.
- Soon the signs and symptoms of suppuration, such as, pain, edema and tenderness increase.
- On the ciliary margin of the lid the orifice of the affected meibomian gland is swollen and enlarged.
- On eversion of the lid yellowish area is seen on tarsal conjunctiva. Preauricular lymph nodes are enlarged and tender.

- Some cases may show general malaise. Sometimes the abscess so formed may burst through the conjunctiva or occasionally it may discharge through the orifice of the gland. It rarely discharges even through the skin.

Complications

- Hordeolum internum may occur in the crop or appearing one after the other over a long period usually when there is a persistent chronic infection in form of chronic conjunctivitis or blepharitis.

- Association of diabetes or debilitating condition favours its appearance in crop or one after the other.

Treatment

- Systemic antibiotic.
- Topical application of antibiotic eye drops six times a day.
- Hot fomentation twice a day.
- Incision and drainage through conjunctiva.
- Improve general health by diet and multi-vitamins.
- Control diabetes and any other focal infection.

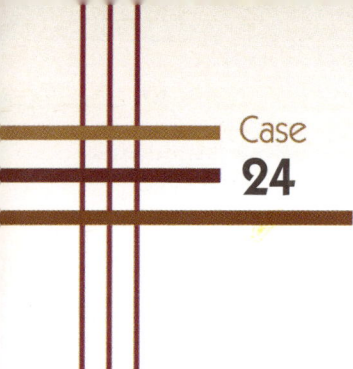
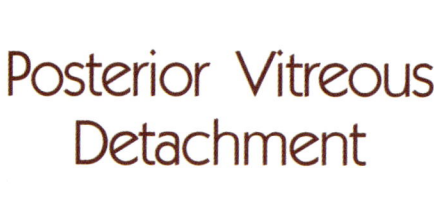

Posterior Vitreous Detachment

Young professional complains of seeing flashes of light in his left eye since two days. Now, he is also seeing large number of floaters before his eye. He is anxious about these symptoms. His working hours are late at night.

External ocular examination is normal.

Visual acuity is normal in both the eyes.

Ophthalmoscopy shows large number of vitreous floaters. Indirect ophthalmoscopy shows posterior detachment of vitreous in left eye.

Diagnosis: Posterior vitreous detachment.

POSTERIOR VITREOUS DETACHMENT

Posterior vitreous detachment is a condition in which there is a separation of the posterior vitreous from the retina (Fig. 24.1).

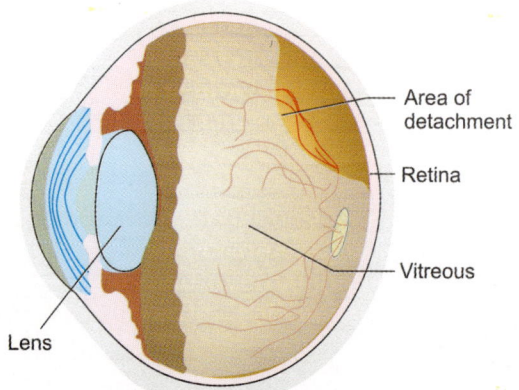

Vitreous detachment

Area of detachment

Retina

Vitreous

Lens

Fig. 24.1: Showing posterior vitreous detachment

Symptoms
- Vitreous floaters
- Photopsia

Vitreous Floaters
- Vitreous floaters appear suddenly and that too in large number that always attracts the attention of the patient. Floaters appear as dark floating spots before the eyes in various shapes and sizes.
- Patient may describe these as per his own observation and comparison to the objects seen in daily life. Thus, some patient will describe these as if fly or mosquito is flying before his eyes. Others may describe these as dark spots, thick or fine, regular or irregular in shape. In some cases vitreous floaters are in the shape of a thread, worm or a cotton wool.
- Floaters are moving freely though his eyes are stationary. The vitreous floaters can be seen by ophthalmoscopy.
- Sudden appearance of large number of floaters must arouse suspicion for posterior detachment of the vitreous.

Photopsia (Flashes of Light)
- Photopsia is yet another important symptom of impending or occurrence of posterior vitreous detachment. The patient complains of perceiving a flash of light as glow or arc streak of light in his field of vision. This perception of flash of light is for very short duration never more than a fraction of a second. This flash of light is visible to him more readily in the dim light or dark surrounding. He

quickly discovers that this flash of light can be elicited readily with the movement of the eyes in the dim illumination or in dark surrounding.

- This phenomenon of flash of light seen by the patient is due to cerebral awareness of vitreous stimulating the retina. This flash of light is commonly seen by the patients who develop syneresis (collapse) of vitreous and in those who have vitreous traction on vitreoretinal lesions.
- Therefore, any patient who complains of photopsia must be thoroughly examined and investigated for vitreoretinal pathology. Photopsia must arouse a suspicion for posterior vitreous detachment unless excluded by examination.

Pathogenesis

- Synchysis and syneresis is an age related phenomenon which occurs universally over the age of sixty-five years usually affecting the upper part of the vitreous.
- The liquefacation and the collapse of vitreous gel can occur due to age or any kind of trival insult to the vitreous that may be in form of mild trauma.
- In some cases hole develops in the thin wall of the posterior vitreous cortex which overlies the fovea. The liquid vitreous passes through this hole into the retro-hyaloid space and forcibly detaches the posterior vitreous surface from the internal limiting membrane of the retina as far as the posterior border of the vitreous base.
- Due to escape of the synchytic fluid the syneresis (collapse) of the posterior vitreous follows thereby the retrohyaloid space is completely filled by the synchytic fluid. This process is known as 'acute rhegmatogenous posterior vitreous detachment with collapse'.
- During this whole process, the patient is likely to see vitreous floaters and photopsia.
- Synchysis senilis is an age related phenomenon giving rise to same symptoms of vitreous floaters and photopsia.
- Therefore, any patient who complains of sudden appearance of floaters and photopsia must be subjected to a thorough examination to exclude retinal breaks, retrovitreal hemorrhage, vitreoretinal traction and posterior vitreous detachment before assigning the age as the causative factor.

Management

- Thorough examination for vitreoretinal pathology.
- If there are lesions then treat them accordingly.
- If there are no lesions then assure the patient that these symptoms are age related due to degeneration of the vitreous, therefore nothing to worry about it. He quickly learns to ignore.
- Any increase in the floaters and appearance of photopsia must be taken seriously and must arouse the suspicion for vitreoretinal pathology.
- Any patient irrespective of age and sex who complains of floaters and photopsia must be subjected to thorough examination at regular intervals.

Quinine Amblyopia

An adult patient enters the clinic helped by two relatives. There is complete loss of vision following treatment for malaria with quinine. He lost the vision following the first single dose.

Ocular examination shows dilated and fixed pupil in both the eyes. Fundus examination shows a cherry spot at the macula with pale disk.

Diagnosis: Quinine amblyopia

QUININE AMBLYOPIA

Quinine amblyopia may follow in susceptible person even with single small dose of 60 mg. Other persons may not have any effect even with high dose. Quinine should not be given more than 150 mg per day.

CILINICAL FEATURES

Visual Acuity

Visual acuity may fall gradually or there may be complete loss of vision in few hours. The vision may be lost to the extent of even absence of perception of light.

Pupil

Both pupils are dilated and immobile. There is no reaction to direct or indirect light.

Fundus

- Optic disk is pale.
- Retinal arteries are extremely attenuated.
- Edema at the macula area.

- Macula shining like cherry giving characteristic picture of cherry red spot resembling to the central retinal artery occlusion (Fig. 25.1).
- Optic disk atrophy follows in due course.
- Pigmentary changes in the periphery.

Prognosis

- Prognosis is poor.
- Some cases may not recover and remain blind.
- Usually, there is some recovery of central vision while peripheral vision is permanently lost providing tubular vision to the patient.
- Recovery may occur in few hours to few days or several weeks so do not see the case as refractory case and so try to treat the patient with all the means.

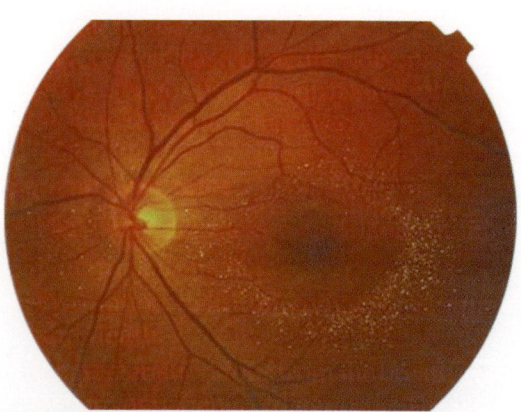

Fig. 25.1: Quinine retinopathy—setting of optic atrophy with cherry red spot at macula

Management

The only treatment is producing vasodilation.

Vasodilation of the central retinal arteries can be achieved by the following means:

- Administration of amyl nitrate.
- Injection of atropine.

- Retrobulbar injection of acetylcholine, and papaverine sulphate.

Following surgical procedures have been suggested:

- Paracentesis of the anterior chamber.
- Filtration surgery.

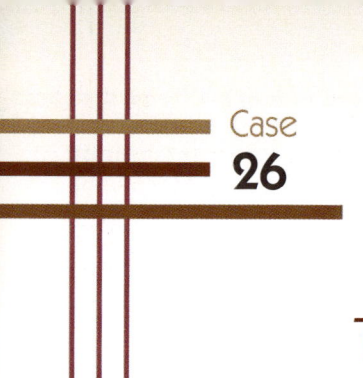

Tobacco Amblyopia

A farmer past fifty enters the clinic with his breath giving a strong smell of stale tobacco. He makes himself comfortable in the chair. He is of a thin built, anxious and shows mild tremors of hand. He complains of weakness, loss of weight, dim vision and associates these to a recent attack of influenza. He has been smoking (*Pipe* or *Chilam*) since his childhood. Since few years he has been drinking alcohol also. His main problem is seeing a mist in front of his eyes.

External ocular examination is normal. Visual acuity in both the eyes is about 6/24.

Fundus examination shows a temporal pallor. There are arteriosclerotic changes in the retinal vessels.

Diagnosis: Tobacco amblyopia

TOBACCO AMBLYOPIA

Tobacco amblyopia is a condition which is characterized by bilateral diminution of the visual acuity with a centro-cecal scotoma.

Tobacco amblyopia is more common if associated with alcoholism and such cases are referred as 'tobacco-alcohol amblyopia'.

CLINICAL FEATURES

Appearance of symptoms range widely. Someone is susceptible while other is immune. The period of smoking also varies. The amount consumed also varies. Usually, there is a history of smoking for years using raw and strong tobacco in pipe or *chilam* to the extent that the odor of breath is of stale tobacco. Further drinking of alcohol potentiates the poison. There is always a history of associated disease; diabetes, influenza, gastric trouble, arteriosclerosis, etc. The patient is usually in the state of ill health, physical depression and under nutrition.

Etiology

Addiction to tobacco.

Its association with drinking alcohol enhances the effect. Tobacco is usually smoked, chewed, snuffed or in inhale while employed in tobacco factory.

Most common mode is pipe smoking with strong tobacco.

Symptoms

- Diminution of visual acuity.
- Difficulty in doing fine work and reading even with spectacle.
- Foggy vision as if there is a mist or a thin grey veil in front of eyes.
- Change in colour values in form of fading.
- An intelligent and romantic patient from a high social status may complain that he feels that the complexion of his wife has changed considerably. He is likely to consult a physician about the change in the complexion of his wife. Physician finding the lady red and rosy, will refer the couple to an eye physician to examine the 'Dear Husband' for his feeling of change in the colour and complexion of his wife. He says emphatically that his wife looks to him greyish rather than reddish, her usual complexion.

Signs

- Patient looks thin, under nourished and physically unfit.
- Breath emits strong odour of stale tobacco.
- Hands may show mild tremors.
- Appears as an anxious and worried person.
- May be in the state of mental depression
- Field charting shows centro-cecal scotoma affecting central vision.
- Fundus shows temporal pallor and may lead to optic atrophy in due course of time (Fig. 26.1).

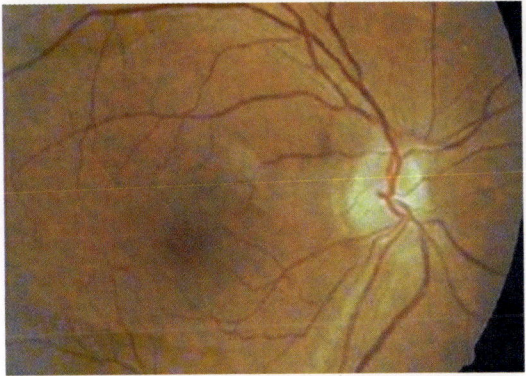

Fig. 26.1: Fundus shows optic atrophy

Management

- Complete abstention from use of tobacco in any form or method.
- Refrain from drinking alcohol.
- Good diet rich in proteins.
- Injection of vitamin B_{12} is very effective.
- Vasodilators are not of much use.

Chloroquine Retinopathy (Bull's Eye Maculopathy)

Young male is on chloroquine therapy for the last one year for rheumatoid arthritis. He complains of blurred vision and a cloudy spot in his field of vision.

External ocular examination is normal.

Visual acuity is 6/12 in both the eyes.

Ophthalmoscopy shows loss of foveal reflex with pigmentation at the macula.

Diagnosis: Bilateral chloroquine retinopathy (Bull's eye maculopathy).

CHLOROQUINE RETINOPATHY

Chloroquine is a synthetic antimalarial drug. It has been used as treatment and for prophylaxis of malaria. Since the discovery of the beneficial use of chloroquine against other disorders it has been widely used for the treatment of lupus erythematosus, rheumatoid arthritis, ankylosing spondylitis, hepatic amebiasis and leishmaniasis. With its wide use for long period reports poured in about its toxicity on the ocular tissues. Involvement of retina leads to visual disturbances with loss of vision (Fig. 27.1).

Symptoms

The usual presenting symptoms of onset of retinopathy are as follows:
- Difficulty in reading.
- Blurring of distant vision.
- Photophobia.
- Photopsia (flashes of light).
- Seeing streaks in front of eyes.
- Cloudy area in the field of vision.

Most of the cases seek the advice of an eye physician soon with any symptom related to visual disorder.

Some cases may remain asymptomatic.

Some cases may report late.

Most of the cases are ignorant about the association of the visual symptoms with

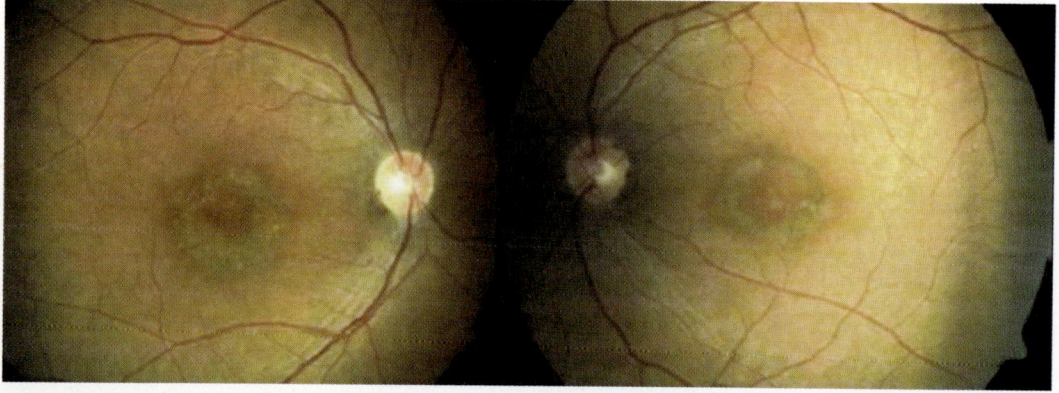

Fig. 27.1: Chloquin neuropathy

intake of chloroquine for their systemic disease unless the treating physician has warned and advised to get the eye check-up at regular intervals of about 6 months.

Signs

The following fundus changes can be seen.

Premaculopathy

- Loss of foveal reflex with mild stippling of macula with pigmentation is lebelled as 'premaculopathy' and the patient is usually asymptomatic.
- Premaculopathy changes are reversible if the intake of the chloroquine is withdrawn.
- Premaculopathy changes are also associated with the aging therefore these must be differentiated from the changes due to drug. Therefore, it becomes necessary to conduct an initial fundus examination and make a note about it for later reference.

Maculopathy

- Macula appears granular with pigmentation surrounded by clear zone of depigmentation.
- This clear zone is again surrounded by another ring of pigmentation.
- Thus, the whole pattern of pigmentation and depigmentation at the macula resembles the bull's-eye of a target used for practice shooting with pistol or rifle.
- These, changes usually continue to progress even after the withdrawal of chloroquine.
- Though the fundus picture is pathognomonic of chloroquine retinopathy yet the fundus picture may vary considerably. Absence of typical maculopathy does not rule out chloroquine intoxication. As some cases shows pigmentary changes in the form of bonecorpuscle pigmentation in the periphery of retina.

CLINICAL INVESTIGATIONS

Fluorescein Angiography

Fluorescein angiography reveals an area around the macula showing leakage. It reveals maculopathy in its early stage.

Visual Fields

- Pericentral or paracentral scotoma. Patient is unable to see the letters at either end of a long word or a sentence. This affects near vision while far vision is normal and unaffected.
- Central scotoma is associated with central loss of vision. Scotoma may extend into the superior temporal quadrant resembling a bitemporal field defect. Further retinal damage may lead to loss of entire visual field.
- It is to be kept in mind that there may be field changes with fundus appearing normal. There may not be any field changes even with changes in the fundus.

Colour Vision

Ishihara pseudoisochromatic plates may demonstrate defect in colour vision most probably due to paracentral scotoma which manifests as difficulty in reading the letters-near vision.

Electroretinography

Changes in electroretinogram confirms retinopathy rather than prognostic test.

PATHOGENESIS

Pathogenesis is the binding of the drug to the intracellular nuclear proteins.

Relationship of the Drug and Retinopathy

- Close relationship of the dose of chloroquine and the period of therapy.
- Total dose of 100 g (about 220 mg per day for 1 year) may be responsible for development of a retinopathy.

- Duration for producing retinopathy varies from 7 months to 10 years of daily dose.
- Therefore, daily dose of 250 mg per day should not be exceeded.
- Regular check-up after every 6 months is essential.
- An initial fundus record is must to know the base line fundus picture.

Management

- No effective treatment for retinopathy.
- Prevent by using the lowest effective dose for that case.
- Withdrawal of drug for short period at intervals will further help to reduce the chances of retinopathy. An initial fundus study followed by study at six monthly intervals is necessary.

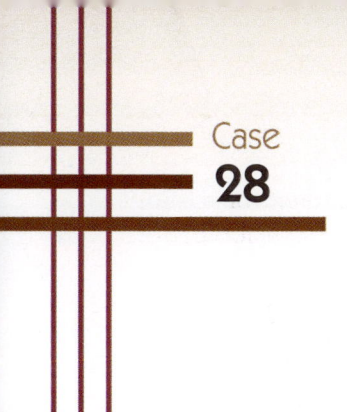

Case
28

Vossius' Ring

Adult young patient attends the clinic with history of injury to his right eye with blunt end of a thick round wooden piece at night. He does not complain of any symptom. He has come for a routine check-up because of the injury.

External examination of the eye is normal. Slit lamp after mydriasis shows a ring of pigment deposited over anterior lens capsule. Fundus is normal.

Diagnosis: Vossius' ring.

VOSSIUS' RING

Vossius' ring is a condition in which the iris pigment is deposited on the anterior lens capsule following a concussion injury to the eye (Fig. 28.1). The size of ring corresponds in size to the pupillary size of that patient.

The Vossius' ring is an imprint of the pupillary border of the iris upon the lens capsule. The imprint occurs at the time of concussion injury in which the iris is suddenly forced against the lens or the lens during rebound strikes against the pupillary aperture of the iris. This also explains the occurrence of duplicate ring of pigment over the lens capsule once when the iris strikes against the lens capsule and second when the lens strikes against the iris.

Vossius' ring is seen only in young people receiving concussion injury. This phenomenon indicates that the iris is capable of depositing the pigment in younger age.

CLINICAL APPEARANCE

The ring of pigment is about 1 mm in breadth and the pigment usually deposit in a single layer. The deposits are tiny brown amorphous granules of pigment derived from the posterior surface of the iris. The size of the ring corresponds to the size of the pupil or it is smaller due to traumatic miosis.

Differential Diagnosis

A Vossius' ring is to be differentiated from the pigment of posterior synechia following iridocyclitis. The pigment left after breaking of the posterior synechia is thick, large and irregular. There is no history of injury and at the same time there are other signs of iridocyclitis.

TREATMENT

As the pigments of Vossius' ring do not affect the vision it does not require any treatment.

Usually, the pigment deposits disappear in due course of time.

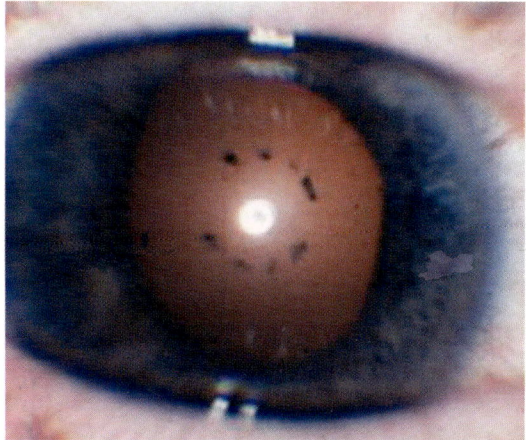

Fig. 28.1: Vossius' ring

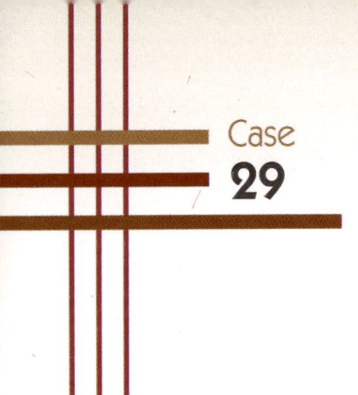

Recurrent Corneal Erosions

A professional rings early in the morning relating the following history:

Doctor, as I woke up, I felt acute pain in my left eye. Now, there is pain, watering, photophobia and foreign body sensation. It is the pain which woke me up.

The history is suggestive of corneal erosion. A history of minor injury to the cornea with the corner of newspaper was confirmed.

Ocular examination with slit lamp shows a minute erosion of the cornea with few grey white spots in the surrounding epithelium.

Diagnosis: Recurrent corneal erosion.

RECURRENT CORNEAL EROSION

Recurrent corneal erosion is a condition in which there is vesiculation of the cornea followed by exfoliation of the epithelium (Fig. 29.1). It is recurrent in cycle for long periods. Usually, there is history of minor corneal abrasion. The common causative

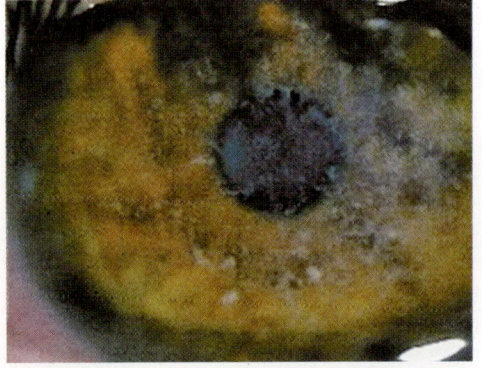

Fig. 29.1: Recurrent corneal erosion

factor is fingernail, corner or edge of newspaper, hanky, etc.

Clinical Presentation

The patient wakes in the morning with an acute pain in the eyes with symptoms of pain, lacrimation, photophobia, mild circumciliary injection and feeling of foreign body sensation.

Clinical Features

- Circum corneal flush.
- One or more minute epithelial bleb or erosion.
- Epithelial filament attached at one end.
- Fluorescein stain is positive.
- Slit lamp shows bleb, erosion or filament with the grey white spots in the loose edematous epithelium.

Pathogenesis

It is due to adherence of the lid to an edematous area of epithelium or a vesicle which is readily torn away on waking up in the morning when the patient opens the lids. There is usually a history of minor trauma of the cornea. This heals quickly but probably irregularly. This results in occurrence of a vesicle which gets torn away on opening of the lids on waking up.

Etiology

Various views are available:
- Minor erosion of the corneal epithelium, passing unnoticed.
- Corneal dystrophy.
- It is neuropathic in nature.
- Hereditary.

The most commonly associated factor is minor erosion of the corneal epithelium. Injury though minor may be acting as trigger mechanism.

Treatment

- Treat the case like any other case of corneal erosion.
- Instillation of antibiotic eyedrops six to eight times a day until the erosion heals and for further 5 days.
- Application of an eye ointment at bedtime until the erosion has healed.
- Instillation of cycloplegic will be helpful.
- Vitamins A and C in high doses for few days shall be helpful for better regeneration of corneal epithelium.
- Some cases may need a chemical cauterisation for proper healing and controlling the recurrences.

Epibulbar Dermoid

Patient presents with a small nodule at the limbus since birth.

On examination, there is a pinkish yellow nodule with dry surface and few hairs.

Diagnosis: Epibulbar dermoid

EPIBULBAR DERMOID

Clinical Features

- Common site for epibulbar dermoid is the limbus in the lower and outer quadrant (Fig. 30.1).
- Usually, it is unilateral. If bilateral then it will place symmetrically in both eyes.

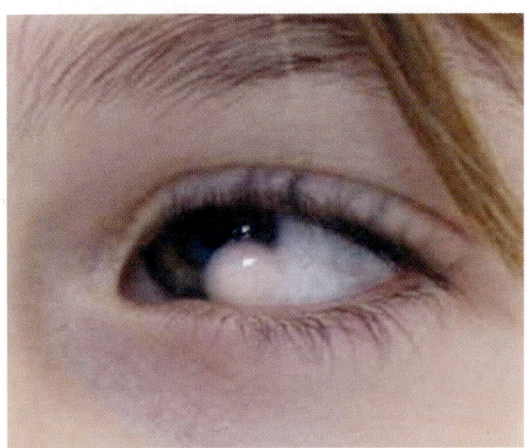

Fig. 30.1: Epibulbar dermoid

- Usually, it appears as round or oval nodule and may be pinkish-yellow in colour.
- Covered with dry conjunctiva and shows few short hairs on its surface.
- Usually, the dermoid is small in size. It may grow slowly and show fast growth at puberty.
- Fixed to the underlying tissue as the deeper layers are continuous with the corneal and scleral tissue.

Dermolipoma

Dermolipoma contains large amount of fatty tissue. These are small yellow tumors of congenital origin, frequently found subconjunctivally. The conjunctiva moves freely over these. Manifest anywhere, near limbus, at the inner angle, or between superior and lateral rectus muscles. These may be multiple. Most of these are of dermoid nature.

Management

Only treatment is the surgical removal of the dermoid. It is better to remove it at an early age and stage before it starts growing at puberty to provide good cosmetic appearance.

Removal in late stage leaves thick scar with cosmetic embarrassment.

Anterior Ring
Staphyloma of Sclera

Patient attends the ophthalmic clinic with complain of bulging bluish-black colored ring all around the black (cornea) of the eye. To begin with this bulging was little and it is gradually increasing in its size. There is mild discomfort due to improper closure of the affected left eye. Ocular examination shows a bluish-black coloured ring of bulged sclera around the limbus in the left eye. The right eye shows bluish coloration around the limbus.

Diagnosis: Anterior ring staphyloma of the sclera.

ANTERIOR RING STAPHYLOMA OF SCLERA

Staphyloma is an ectatic condition of the sclera in which the uveal tissue is incarcerated (Fig. 31.1). It occurs in a situation where the sclera is weak by the passage of blood vessels. Anteriorly in the region of ciliary body, the sclera is pierced by many vessels which enters and leave the eye. The main vessels are anterior ciliary arteries and veins. This area is further weakened by the presence of canal of Schlemm. This weakness of the sclera in the ciliary region and associated high intraocular pressure play part in the development of an anterior ring staphyloma of the sclera in the ciliary region.

1. LOCALIZED ANTERIOR STAPHYLOMA

A localized anterior scleral staphyloma (Fig. 31.2) develops at the site of disease process in the ciliary region such as:

- Scleritis and episcleritis
- Tuberculoma
- Uveitis
- Endarteritis
- Trauma.

A localized anterior scleral staphyloma remains localized at the site. It has been further divided into two types.

Ciliary Staphyloma

It occurs in the region of ciliary body wherein the anterior ciliary arteries have passage and emerge at the anterior border of the bulge. In the ciliary staphyloma, the dark striae of the ciliary processes can be seen on transillumination.

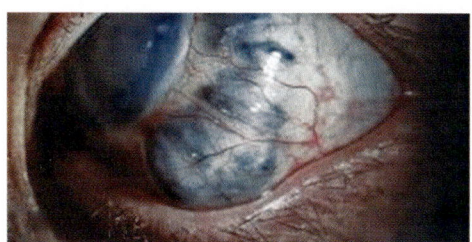

Fig. 31.1: Ring staphyloma

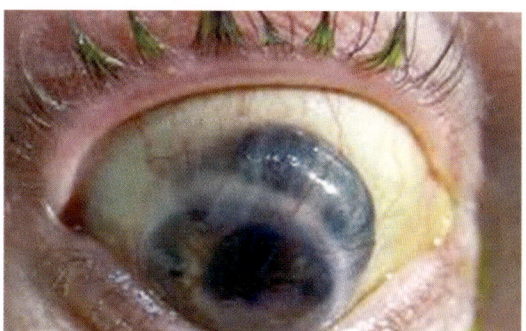

Fig. 31.2: Localized anterior staphyloma

Intercalary Staphyloma

It occurs between the anterior extremity of the ciliary body and the limbus. Here, the sclera is weak due to passage of anterior ciliary veins and canal of Schlemm.

The ciliary and intercalary staphylomas can be differentiated by the fact that, in the ciliary staphyloma the anterior ciliary arteries emerge at the anterior border of the bulge, while in the intercalary staphyloma these emerge posteriorly.

2. CLINICAL FEATURES AND MANAGEMENT

An anterior staphyloma is a progressive lesion. With the time, the bulge increases and other parts of the eye get involved in form of atrophy of uveal tissue, iridodialysis, luxation of lens and even involvement of the cornea.

The whole eyeball looks very big due to bulge all round the cornea.

The margins are sharp and it appears lobulated.

It can be dimpled when touched.

There is discomfort due to improper closure of the eye by lids.

The eye is likely to develop exposure keratitis.

There is pain that is associated with rise of intraocular pressure.

If not taken care of then the ultimate result is rupture of the globe and all the complications associated with rupture.

Management

As the bulge is due to weak sclera associated with high intraocular pressure. Therefore, the best and early line of treatment is to perform surgery to reduce intraocular pressure. If the pressure is controlled, most likely the bulge will remain stationary or may even reduce in its size. Scleroplasty has been suggested.

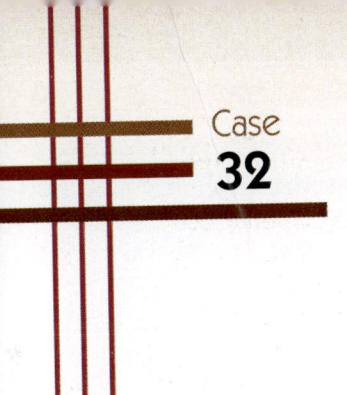

Luxation of Lens

A n elderly farmer complains of severe pain in his right eye following a mild trauma with tail of buffalo while milking.

Ocular examination shows circumciliary congestion with whitish pale nuclear lens in anterior chamber.

Diagnosis: Dislocation of lens in anterior chamber.

LUXATION OF LENS

Luxation (dislocation) of the lens is a condition in which the lens is completely displaced from the patellar fossa. The lens may be displaced at the following sites:

- Remains incarcerated (hanging) in the pupil.
- In the anterior chamber.
- In the liquid vitreous as floater or fixed to ciliary body or retina.
- In the subretinal or subscleral space.
- Subconjunctival dislocation of the lens or thrown out of eye.

Etiology

Congenital Factor

The lens may be subluxated as ectopia lentis as seen in Marfan's and Marchesani's syndromes. Even a mild trauma is enough to displace the lens completely from the patellar fossa. The subluxation is due to defective zonules in one sector.

Trauma

It plays an important role in the displacement of a lens. A severe trauma may even displace a normal lens with normal zonular fibres.

Even a mild trauma may displace a mature or hypermature lens. In these cases the zonules have degenerated due to ageing.

Consecutive or Spontaneous

Main factors involved

- Degeneration or atrophy of zonular fibres.
- Degeneration and liquefaction of the vitreous gel.

These two factors are commonly seen in cases of high myopia, choroiditis, cyclitis, detachment of retina or simple senile degeneration.

Other factor favouring

- Hypermaturity of the cataractous lens.
- Degeneration of zonular fibres with stretching.

These two factors combined favours spontaneous dislocation of a hypermature lens with a mild trauma which may even pass unnoticed or does not attract attention until it is complicated by the secondary glaucoma or uveitis.

Because of this readiness of the lens to dislocate it is advisable that patient should not be allowed to make his lens a hypermature lens. In a case of hypermature lens, one can elicit the tremulousness of the lens as well as of the iris. This is due to shrinkage of the lens and rupture of few fibres of zonule due to degeneration.

CLINICAL FEATURES AND MANAGEMENT

1. LENS INCARCERATED (HANGING) IN THE PUPILLARY AREA

This occurs following a trauma. It is a rare event in which the lens suffers an axial rotation of 90° so that the equator of the lens presents in the pupillary area. Probably a spasmodic contraction of the pupil may have played a part in engagement of the lens in the pupil in this position. The lens may maintain this position or usually it shall dislocate either in the anterior chamber or vitreous.

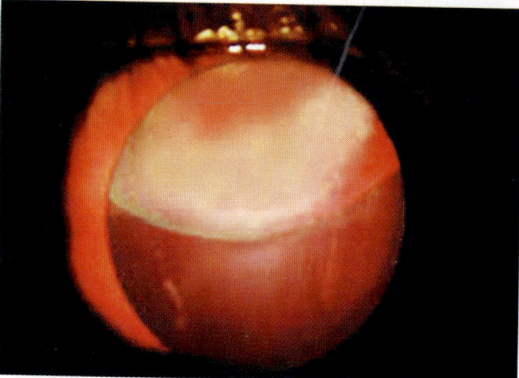

Fig. 32.2: Luxation of lens upper part

2. DISLOCATION IN THE ANTERIOR CHAMBER

A clear lens dislocated into the anterior chamber gives a characteristic appearance (Fig. 32.1).

- Lens looks like a drop of oil placed in the anterior chamber. Its peripheral rim gives a golden luster. The iris is clearly visible through the lens. The pupil is spasmodically constricted.
- Cataractous or an opaque lens appears as a white pale globular disk in the anterior chamber. The lens usually turns completely so that the posterior surface of the lens is towards the cornea.

The lens in its anterior dislocation position, whether clear or opaque may sometimes be well-tolerated (Fig. 32.2). Usually, the hyper-mature lens disintegrates and ruptures filling the anterior chamber with fluid liquid which may absorb slowly.

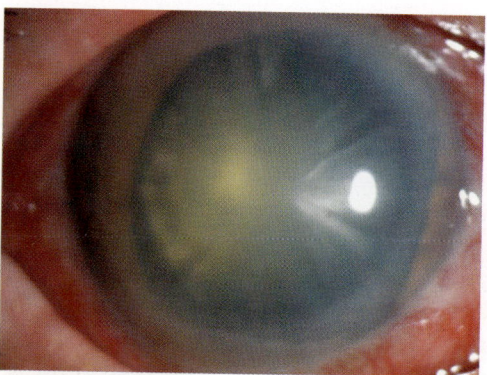

Fig. 32.1: Dislocation in anterior chamber

Most frequently the dislocated lens in the anterior chamber produces the following complications:

- *Corneal dystrophy/opacity:* The lens present in the anterior chamber comes in contact with the endothelial surface of the cornea repeatedly. This repeated contact leads to corneal dystrophy or opacity.
- *Secondary glaucoma:* Secondary glaucoma occurs due to blockage of the circulation of the aqueous humour from the pupil and at the angle of the anterior chamber.
- *Iridocyclitis:* Iridocyclitis sets in due to constant irritation of iris and ciliary body.

Management

Removal of the lens at an early stage is the best treatment to avoid all the above mentioned three intractable complications which usually results in the loss of vision.

3. DISLOCATION IN THE VITREOUS

Clinically the dislocation of lens in the vitreous (posterior dislocation) produces the following picture:

- Anterior chamber is deep.
- Iris is tremulous.
- Pupil appears jet black.
- Lens can be seen by ophthalmoscopy.
- Lens may be clear or opaque.

If the vitreous is healthy the lens appears to be afloat in the anterior vitreous near the ciliary body. This lens may show some movements with the movements of the eye. Gradually, the lens becomes anchored or attached due to organized bands or membranes.

Clear and intact lens is well-tolerated by the eye. It may remain quiet without causing any complications for years until it becomes opaque or excites the ciliary body with which it is usually attached.

Rupture of the lens capsule whether the lens is clear or cataractous allows the proteins to escape. This excites a phacotoxic uveitis.

Wandering Lens

The lens may move about freely in the liquified vitreous. Thus, the lens can move with the movement of the eye. Ultimately, it gets fixed to retina somewhere usually in the lower part.

Cases have been observed in which it moves between the anterior vitreous and anterior chamber.

Subretinal or Subscleral Dislocation of the Lens

The lens may become subretinal if it slips through the retinal tear.

It may insert itself between the sclera and ciliary body to become subscleral.

Subconjunctival Dislocation of the Lens or thrown out

It occurs after contusion injury to the eyeball in which there is scleral rupture. In such cases the lens may completely be thrown out of the eye or it may lie under the conjunctiva.

4. COMPLICATIONS OF DISLOCATION OF THE LENS

Uveitis

Uveitis is the common complication following a dislocation of the lens. The dislocated lens can cause uveitis due to constant irritation of the ciliary body, if the lens is resting or attached to the ciliary body. Phaco-anaphylactic uveitis follows with a hypermature lens dislocation. Both types of uveitis causes an increase in the intraocular pressure.

Secondary glaucoma

Secondary glaucoma always follows the dislocation of the lens. It can occur due to the following factors:

- Block at the pupil by the lens or the vitreous.
- Block at the angle of the anterior chamber due to peripheral anterior synechia.
- Phacolytic glaucoma
- Angle recession glaucoma.
- Hypertensive glaucoma following uveitis.
- Glaucoma is more common with anterior dislocation of the lens than posterior dislocation of the lens.
- Glaucoma is more common with dislocation of a hypermature cataractous lens than a clear lens.

Retinal detachment

Retinal detachment is one of the worst complication following a dislocation of the lens. The dislocation makes it difficult to examine and locate the retinal tear and treat it.

Corneal dystrophy or opacity

It is seen in cases with dislocation of the lens in the anterior chamber. The lens in the chamber constantly rubs against the endothelial surface and thereby results in the development of opacity or dystrophy.

Management

Dislocated lens may remain quiet for years without causing any symptom or complication. Thus, it was thought that such lens should be left alone until they produce symptoms or complications.

The patient may not be able to reach the eye surgeon when the dislocated lens shall give rise to symptoms and complications. Thus, the best treatment of a dislocated lens is surgical removal with the first opportunity without waiting for manifestation of symptoms and complications.

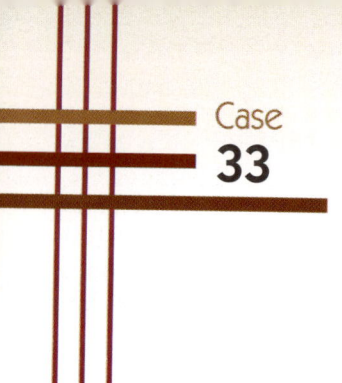

Temporal Arteritis

An elderly male complains of pain in the left temporal region and shoulder girdle since two months. There is also associated loss of vision in his left eye. Even simple combing excites pain in the scalp.

Ocular examination show visual acuity in his right eye 6/6 and left eye 6/24.

Ophthalmoscopy shows optic atrophy with cupping. Intraocular pressure is normal.

Diagnosis: *Temporal arteritis*

TEMPORAL ARTERITIS

Few cases of anterior ischemic optic neuropathy do not show typical systemic manifestations. In these cases the diagnosis becomes difficult and one has to rely on few important clinical signs and symptoms and laboratory investigations. The most common cause for anterior ischemic optic neuropathy is 'atherosclerosis'. The next common cause is 'giant cell arteritis'.

Clinical Picture

- There is loss of vision in the affected eye. Sometimes both the eyes are involved.
- Few cases present with pain in the temporal region.
- Others may complain of headache which may be generalized or localized to frontal, occipital or temporal areas.
- If headache is the presenting symptom, then it can be very severe. Patient seeks advice of an eye physician because of his headache.
- Few cases present with tenderness in the scalp. The tenderness is so acute that even

the blowing of a fan wind or combing the hair excites pain in the scalp.

- Patient may complain of pain in the shoulder girdle. It disturbs him for his own routine work of dressing or driving, etc.
- Some cases may not present any of the systemic manifestations. The only complain is the loss of vision. These cases have been labelled as cases of *occult temporal arteritis*.

Clinical Signs

- On palpation of the temporal artery it may be tender, inflamed and nodular (Fig. 33.1). It feels like a hard cord.
- It cannot be flattened against the bones of temple region.
- Few cases may show a normal temporal artery. Although the artery appears normal to feel yet it shows typical histopathological changes on biopsy.

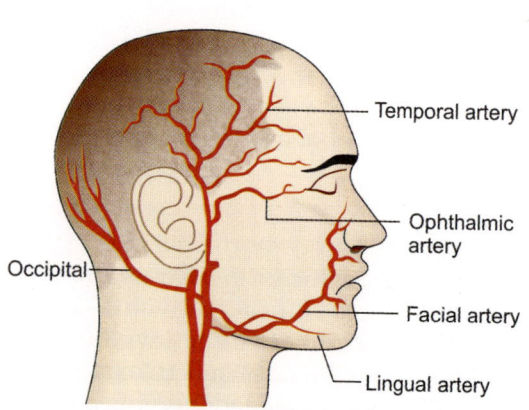

Fig. 33.1: Temporal artery

- Visual acuity is subnormal.
- Visual fields are impaired.
- Ophthalmoscopy show optic atrophy with or without cupping.
- Optic atrophy may set in late due to posterior ischemic optic neuropathy.

Investigations

1. *Erythrocyte sedimentation rate*: Erythrocyte sedimentation rate (ESR) is very high usually above 100 mm/h or more. One must remember that the erythrocyte sedimentation rate is high in elderly about 40 mm/h. Some cases may show a normal erythrocyte sedimentation rate yet the biopsy of the temporal artery is positive.
2. *C-reactive protein*: The C-reactive protein is invariably raised. It is helpful in the cases with normal erythrocyte sedimentation rate.
3. *Temporal artery biopsy*: Biopsy of the temporal artery is confirmatory. Yet there are cases in whom even after taking a biopsy of about 2.5 cm of the artery the changes are not seen. This is due to variation in the extent of the involvement of the artery. The part taken for biopsy may have escaped the changes.

Diagnosis

Diagnosis primarily bases on the clinical signs and symptoms. Loss of vision and Optic atrophy is diagnostic. Increased erythrocyte sedimentation rate or C-reactive protein further confirms it.

Treatment

The only treatment is steroids in full doses to begin with and taper off every week and thus gradually bring to maintenance dose daily. This minimum dose of steroids may be required for long-time. Erythrocyte sedimentation rate may help and guide if it was raised before starting the steroids.

Subconjunctival Ecchymosis

An elderly male patient past sixties enters the clinic with anxiety and points towards the red patch in his right eye which was noticed by his wife today morning soon after he came out of toilet and sat down for a morning cup of tea.

Ocular examination shows small patch of subconjunctival hemorrhage on the outer bulbar conjunctiva.

Diagnosis: Subconjunctival ecchymosis

SUBCONJUNCTIVAL ECCHYMOSIS

Subconjunctival ecchymosis is seen commonly in elderly persons and it varies in degree from a small patch to a large patch reaching to the limbus and sometimes even covering the lower fornix.

Ecchymosis occur frequently in the exposed part of the bulbar conjunctiva where even small leakage of blood finds space in the loose meshes of the connective tissue manifesting as fairly large amount of blood leak.

Sudden appearance of red eye alarms and forces the patient to consult ophthalmologist immediately. Sudden appearance of subconjunctival hemorrhage is alarming for general systemic check-up for hypertension and diabetes. A small patch of subconjunctival hemorrhage shall take about two weeks to get completely absorbed.

Topical instillation of soothing eyedrops helps to provide mental relief to the patient.

CLINICAL FEATURES AND MANAGEMENT

Etiology

1. Local Trauma to the Eye

Local minor trauma is the most common cause for subconjunctival ecchymosis. Sometimes even rubbing the eyes to get relief from itching can cause ecchymosis.

2. Petechial Hemorrhage in Conjunctivitis

Petechial hemorrhages are commonly seen in any acute conjunctivitis. It is more common with pneumococcal conjunctivitis.

3. In Children with Whooping Cough

Large amount of subconjunctival ecchymosis has been observed in children with whooping cough. In fact, the child is brought to the eye clinic for subconjunctival hemorrhage. It is the ophthalmologist who directs the parents to get the child treated for whooping cough. Parents fail to understand how cough can be associated with hemorrhage in the eyes.

Subconjunctival hemorrhage in children due to whooping cough is usually bilateral and profuse even to the extent to force out the lower fornices (Fig. 34.1).

Subconjunctival ecchymosis is also seen in some children soon after violent bout of vomiting.

Pathogenesis for subconjunctival hemorrhage in whooping cough and following vomiting is sudden and severe venous congestion of the head.

4. Systemic Vascular and Metabolic Diseases

An elderly patient with arteriosclerosis, hypertension and diabetes can get a patch

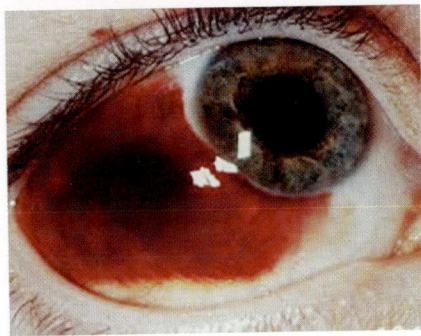

Fig. 34.1: Subconjunctival hemorrhage

of small subconjunctival hemorrhage even with mild physical strain at the stools or force to push or lift heavy objects. Fragile arterioles of the conjunctiva give way due to increased venous pressure.

5. Other Rare Causes

i. Severe venous congestion of head and thorax

Subconjunctival ecchymosis has been seen in the persons who are engaged in the profession wherein they need to blow out, e.g. workers in glass factory, blowing the trumpet.

It has been observed in persons suffering from fits.

It is seen after strangulation in cases that get crushed during stampede and in accidents.

In all these cases the pathogenesis is sudden and severe increase in venous congestion and pressure.

ii. Hemorrhagic purpura

These include thrombocytopenic purpura, vascular purpura, thrombocytopenia, leukemia and anemia.

iii. Injury to orbital structures

- *In fracture of the roof of the orbit*: The blood tracks along the levator muscle to upper fornix and lids.
- *In fracture of the floor of the orbit*: The blood tracks along lower fornix to lids.
- *In fracture of the apex of the orbit*: The blood tracks along the lateral rectus muscle to bulbar conjunctiva.
- *In fracture of the orbital plate of sphenoid*: the blood tracks along the temporal aspect of the globe and then to conjunctiva.

- *In fracture of the base of the skull*: The blood tracks along the floor of the orbit to fornix and conjunctiva.

Usually, it takes 12 to 24 hours for the blood to reach the subconjunctival tissue.

iv. Local vascular anomaly

Subconjunctival hemorrhage may result from an angiomal tumor, varicosity, aneurysm and telangiectasis.

v. Acute febrile systemic infections

Petechial spots may be seen in cases that have fever due to influenza, measles, typhoid, diphtheria, malaria and septicemia.

vi. Unknown

Cases have been seen without any apparent cause.

Clinical Investigation

- Complete systemic check-up.
- Complete cardiovascular check-up.

Laboratory Investigations

- Complete blood picture
- Platelet count.
- Blood sugar—fasting and post-prandial.
- Any other test as required.

Management

- Assure the patient that it is common and insignificant.
- If the fornices are involved then apply cold packs over closed lids twice a day for two days.
- If fornices are forced out then evacuate the blood by simple small nick in the conjunctiva. The blood flows out. Little pressure on the swollen conjunctiva will further help the blood to flow out easily.
- Instillation of soothing eyedrops four times a day if the patch is small.
- Instillation of antibiotic eyedrops if there is large amount of blood involving fornices.
- Ask the patient to report soon if there is any increase in the area of hemorrhage.
- Assure that even a small patch takes about 2 to 3 weeks to get completely absorbed.

Capillary Angioma of Left Lid and Face

Young mother enters the clinic with her newborn baby about one year of age. She points towards the peculiar and conspicuous dark red areas covering the left lid and face.

Ocular examination shows areas of port wine stains over the left upper lid and left side of face. On palpation these stains are not compressible.

Diagnosis: Capillary angioma of left lid and face (Fig. 35.1).

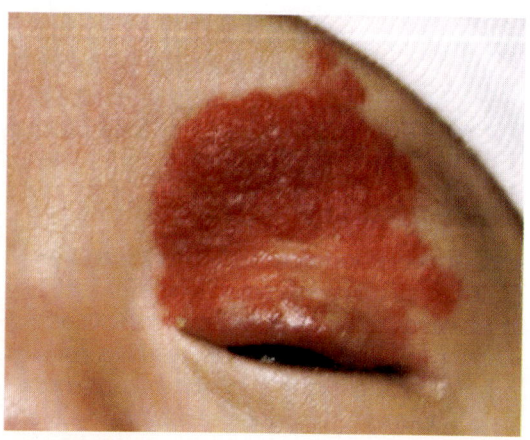

Fig. 35.1: Capillary angioma lid and face

CAPILLARY ANGIOMA OF LEFT LID AND FACE

1. PORT WINE STAINS

Capillary angiomas are the most common form of hemangiomas seen clinically. These appear as dark red slightly elevated areas covering variable part of the lid and face. It involves the area covered by distribution of one or more branches of the fifth nerve. Thus, it may affect only a small area of one lid or may cover large area of the face or even the entire area of fifth nerve.

Pathologically the capillary angioma is made-up of very superficial dilated capillaries with little connective tissue stroma. Capillary angioma is stationary. It is cosmetic embarrassment.

2. STRAWBERRY MARK

A capillary angioma with strawberry mark is also seen. It consists of one or more bright red, soft and globular masses like strawberry. These arise shortly after birth and increase in size for a few months and then regress spontaneously within few years.

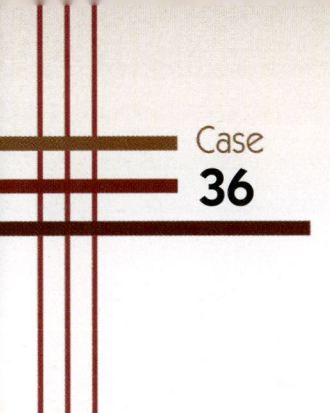

Ecchymosis of Lids

Patient attends the ophthalmic clinic with his left eye covered with hanky and palm of his left hand with history of concussion injury few hours ago.

Ocular examination shows markedly swollen left black lid. On retraction of the lid the underlying eyeball is normal with extensive subconjunctival ecchymosis.

Diagnosis: Ecchymosis of lid and conjunctiva.

ECCHYMOSIS OF LIDS

- Most common cause for ecchymosis of the lid is concussion injury. The blood tends to diffuse through the loose connective tissue of the lid.
- Lid become tense and swollen as the blood collects in the connective tissue of the lid only.
- Spread of blood to forehead is checked by the firm adhesion of the fascia at the eyebrow.
- Spread of blood to cheek is checked by the firm adhesion to the naso-jugal fold.
- Spread of the blood to the upper lip is checked by the firm adhesion at the naso-malar fold.
- Due to these firm adhesions the lids get enormously swollen closing the eye completely. The upper lid may overhang the lower lid.
- On the day of the injury the left eye (injured side) gets swollen and tense.
- On second day the patient and relations get worried due to observation of the swelling spreading to the opposite lid also.

This swelling of the opposite lid is due to crossing over of the blood from the injured left lid to the opposite upper lid and later even to the lower also.

- This crossing of the blood from the eyelid of one eye to the eylid of the opposite eye occurs across the nasal bridge. The skin of the nasal bridge is thick therefore the continuity of the black eye is not visible to the observer. This is the cause of worry for patient and relatives.
- Explain this phenomenon to the patient and relatives to give them mental relief that this is natural process to diffuse the blood early.
- With ecchymosis of the lid the ecchymosis of the conjunctiva is invariably present in minor or major degree.
- Ecchymosis of the conjunctiva can occur without ecchymosis of the lid. Even a minor trauma to the conjunctiva can cause subconjunctiva ecchymosis.

CLINICAL FEATURES AND MANAGEMENT

Lid of the injured side is swollen and tense.

Swelling may cause the upper lid to overhang the lower lid (Fig. 36.1).

Eyeball is completely closed by swollen lid. One may need lid retractors to examine the eyeball.

Ecchymosis of the conjunctiva may be minor or large covering the whole bulbar conjunctiva and even lower fornix that may bulge out.

Cornea is normal.

Pupillary reaction is normal.

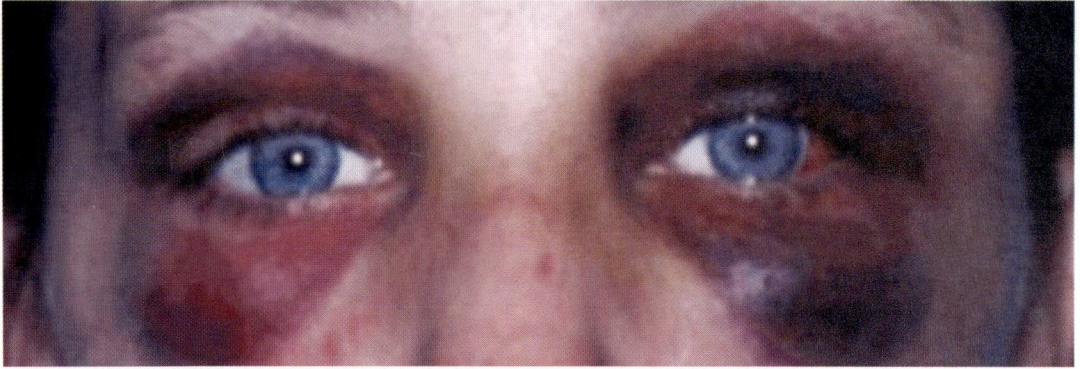

Fig. 36.1: Ecchymosis both lids and conjunctiva with clear nose bridge

Ocular movements may show restriction and pain.

Ophthalmoscopy shows normal fundus.

Management

The first thing is to examine the eyeball and thereafter assure the patient and relatives that as far as the eye is concerned there is nothing to worry.

If the ecchymosis of the injured eye is large causing both the lids to swell and cover the eye then warn the patient and relatives that they may see the black lid of the opposite eye in a day or so due to diffusion of blood from injured side to the opposite side. It is a natural process to absorb the blood early by diffusion.

Ice-packs—three times a day for 4–6 days.

Systemic antibiotic is must as a prophylaxis against infection of the hematoma.

Topical antibiotic eye drops 4 times and eye ointment at bedtime.

Explain the patient that it shall take at least three weeks for complete absorption of blood.

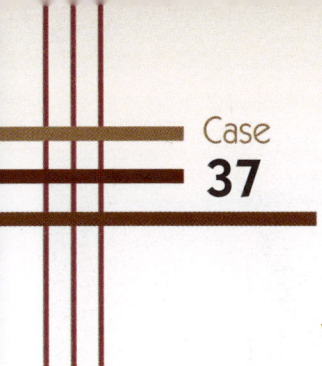

Vitreous Hemorrhage

Young adult male complains of seeing everything red for short-time and thereafter there was complete loss of vision. There is no history of trauma or any disease known to him.

External ocular examination is normal.

Visual acuity in his affected eye is just hand movements. Visual acuity in his other eye is normal 6/6.

Ophthalmoscopy shows no red reflex. Only faint glow is visible in the periphery.

Diagnosis: Vitreous hemorrhage

VITREOUS HEMORRHAGE

Etiology

- Etiology of the vitreous hemorrhage is not in the vitreous gel itself but outside the gel.
- Vitreous hemorrhage occurs due to degenerative, inflammatory or neoplastic diseases of the retina and choroid.
- Trauma plays an important role.

1. Retinal Tear

Retinal tear due to contraction and detachment of the vitreous is the most common cause for vitreous hemorrhage. Most common in the posterior detachment of the vitreous.

Vitreous strand can tear the retina producing a horse shoe tear or hole. Thus, a case presenting with a sudden appearance of vitreous hemorrhage should be thoroughly subjected to locate tear or hole in the retina.

2. Vascular Diseases of the Retina

The most common conditions are diabetic retinopathy, hypertensive retinopathy, Eales's disease and occlusion of the central retinal vein. Ophthalmoscopic examination of the opposite eye leads to diagnosis.

3. Hemopoietic Diseases

The common diseases are anemia, leukemia and purpura.

4. Retinitis Proliferans

Cases with retinitis proliferans are likely to suffer from vitreous hemorrhage. Here again the examination of the opposite eye helps in clinching the diagnosis.

5. Trauma

It is also one of the common causes for vitreous hemorrhage. It can be trigger for a diseased retina or retinal vessel.

Symptoms

- An intelligent person can see and remember seeing red vision prior to complete loss of vision from vitreous hemorrhage. Vision reduces to hand movements.
- Some cases may complain of photopsia and floaters prior to loss of vision. The symptom of photopsia and floaters is due to posterior detachment of the vitreous which is again the most common cause for vitreous hemorrhage.

Signs

- Anterior segment is normal.
- No red reflex on ophthalmoscopy. There may be a faint glow from periphery or on movement of the eye which may displace the clot.

- Slit lamp shows red blood cells and debris behind the lens and in the anterior vitreous.

Course and Prognosis

- Massive hemorrhage in the vitreous tends to diffuse anteriorly and centrally therefore it results in great loss of vision reducing to hand movement.
- Hemorrhage in the healthy vitreous shows finger like projections in the vitreous from the site of bleeding. The blood moves forward along the vitreous fibres.
- Hemorrhage in healthy vitreous clots early and takes a longer time to resolve therefore the patient takes long-time to show improvement in his visual acuity.
- Hemorrhage in liquified degenerated vitreous with lacuna in the vitreous appears like subhyaloid hemorrhage (Fig. 37.1). It resolves early showing improvement in the visual acuity.
- Prognosis is good as most cases show resolution of vitreous hemorrhage.

Management

- Complete bedrest with head end of the bed elevated so that the blood in the vitreous shall settle down minimizing the dispersion in the vitreous. In a day or two the upper part of the fundus may be visible on ophthalmoscopy to locate any tear or a hole in the retina. This shall help the surgeon to manage accordingly.

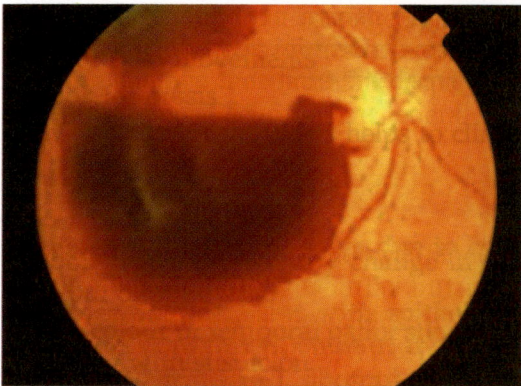

Fig. 37.1: Vitreous hemorrhage—subhyaloid

- Re-examine the patient after complete rest for one week. If there is no tendency for resolution of the vitreous hemorrhage assessed by the reflex of fundus then make him ambulatory. He should be examined every two weeks or so on follow-up.
- Vitrectomy is indicated if the blood does not clear up and if the visual acuity is less than 6/60 with normal electroretinogram and ultrasonography.
- Photocoagulation is indicated if the vitreous hemorrhage is due to occlusion of the central retinal vien.
- Case with Eales' disease needs medical therapy, laser therapy and vitrectomy.

The most important part in the treatment is the rest and diagnosis of the condition which has resulted in occurrence of vitreous hemorrhage and examination of the opposite eye to diagnose any systemic disease responsible for vitreous hemorrhage.

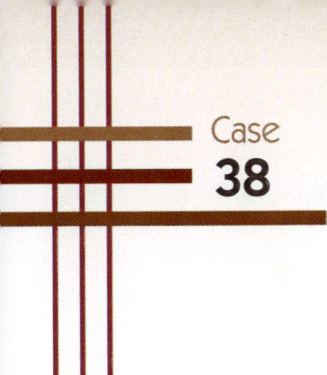

Solar Photophthalmia

Young boy in teens complains of dazzling sensation. There is a history of looking at the sun eclipse five days earlier. Since then there is an annoying after image of the sun eclipse visible to him.

Diagnosis: Eclipse blindness.

1. ECLIPSE BLINDNESS

Eclipse blindness is produced after looking at the sun during the eclipse phase. Blindness due to looking at the sun is known for a very long period. Normally, humans can look at the sun only for a fraction of a second. During sun eclipse humans can look at the sun for long period without any glare. The effect on the eyes varies with the time of exposure.

Patient may perceive only after-image on minimal exposure for few days.

Patient's central vision is affected on long exposure.

Eyes Involved

Usually, it is the involvement of both the eyes as person looks at the sun eclipse by both the eyes open.

It may be unilateral if the person is using inadequate protective glass. In this case he closes the left eye and looks at the eclipse by the dominant right eye.

Varying Effect

The effect of watching eclipse varies with the following factors:
- Degree of pigmentation of the fundus of an individual.
- Refractive state of the eye. Myope may escape.

- Watching for long period is more effective than watching intermittently.
- Climatic condition plays an importent role. Clear weather is more harmful than cloudy weather.
- Young people get afflicted more than oldys. Probably the transmission of light through the lens plays some role.
- An aphakic eye gets afflicted more than normal eye.

Symptoms

Patients may complain of the following subjective symptoms depending on their observation and expression:
- Dazzling sensation
- After-image of the sun eclipse
- Photophobia
- Photopsia
- Chromatopsia (red, yellow or blue vision)
- Scotoma light or dark
- Blurring of vision
- Distortion of the objects
- Any other symptom related to vision
- Most common symptom is blurred vision, as if seeing through a veil and vision reduced to about 6/24–18.

Ophthalmoscopic Picture
- Fundus may appear normal.
- Macular area may appear darker than usual.
- Edema at the macula with dull or absent foveal reflex. Circular light reflex from the border of the edematous macula.

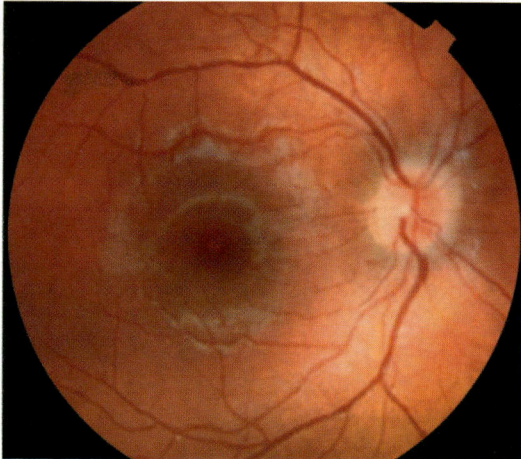

Fig. 38.1: Solar retinitis—edema at macula

- Pigmentary changes at the macula with dark or few yellow white spots.
- Macular cyst.
- Macular hole.

Course

Most cases with minimal affection pay no attention to the early disturbances of vision. Most of these cases improves within a month and lead a normal life. The minimal loss of vision is not noticed by them. It is only on routine examination the eye physician may find changes at the macula with reduced visual acuity. On asking about the history of looking at the eclipse quite often it is positive. Though the eye physician puts the blame to eclipse but the patient puts the blame to some minor trauma which everyone is likely to suffer.

Management

- An early case reporting within few days needs treatment though however minor may be his symptom and fundus changes.
- Short course of systemic steroids.
- A delayed case discovered on routine examination of fundus needs no treatment for the changes at the macula and associated loss of some visual acuity.
- Some cases may show some improvement with glasses.

2. SNOW BLINDNESS

Any person who happens to look at the dazzling reflection of sufficient intensity from a surface of large extensity, such as sea, desert, snow or ice field, for long hours is likely to develop the symptoms of photophthalmia. As solar photophthalmia is encountered more on snow therefore it has acquired a popular title as 'snow blindness'. Any amateur mountaineer at high altitudes can suffer from snow blindness if not using protective glasses.

Snow Blindness

The most common and acute form of snow blindness is seen after exposure to bright sunlight on a snowfield or snow mountain. The term, snow blindness is a misnomer. The photophthalmia is not caused by snow or any other reflecting surface such as sea and desert but by the solar energy reflected from these large surfaces of high reflectivity. Further, the person does not become blind but develops the symptoms of photophthalmia.

Symptoms of Photophthalmia

The symptoms vary with the intensity and duration of exposure.

Further, there is a varying latent period again depending upon the intensity and duration of exposure to reflected solar energy. The latent period can be as short as 30 minutes or as long as about 12 to 24 hours after exposure.

A typical case with moderate exposure will have the following symptoms:

- To begin with there is slight pricking sensation, followed by foreign body sensation as if the eye is full of sand particles. Followed with pain associated with photophobia, lacrimation and marked blepharospasm.
- These symptoms are on peak by midnight, making the patient miserable.
- Patient is in agony with slightest attempt to open the eyes or even putting on the ordinary home light.

By the time, the patient attends the ophthalmic clinic the objective signs have appeared. Thus, the objective signs follow subjective symptoms.

Signs of Snow Blindness

- Lids are swollen and edematous.
- Conjunctiva is intensely congested with chemosis.
- Cornea is denuded of epithelium entirely or at isolated places.
- Fluorescein stain is positive.
- Pupil is miotic.

The eyes can only be examined after proper topical anesthesia.

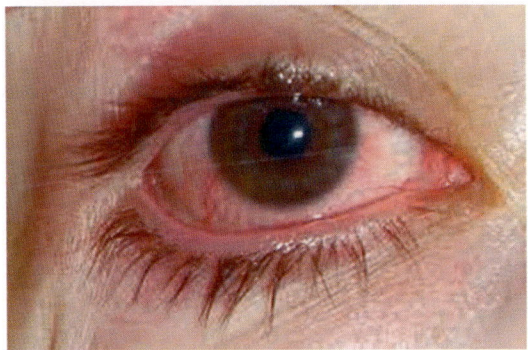

Fig. 38.2: Eye exposed to large surface of snow

Course and Prophylaxis

- Acute symptoms are on peak for 12 to 24 hours and thereafter the discomfort starts showing decline in its intensity and symptoms disappear in 2 to 4 days.
- Some photophobia and congestion of the eyes persists for few more days.
- Patient must be advised not to expose himself again at least for a further period of one month or so or wear protective goggles with sidepieces.
- Usually, a short exposure does not produce any kind of symptoms. That is why the person who is exposed becomes careless. Patient should be advised that the short exposures are additive within a period of 24 hours and are therefore harmful. The person must use protective goggles all the time howsoever short it may be to save self from acute subjective agony of solar photophthalmia.

Management

- Topical Antibiotic eyedrops to prevent infection.
- Topical Atropine, one drop daily gives relief from ciliary neuralgia.
- Bandage with cold compresses gives some relief.

The best plan to provide relief from acute agony of pain is to give him strong analgesic and sedative. If he can be provided relief for 12 to 24 hours, it is gratifying. Thereafter, the distressing symptoms reduce in intensity.

Industrial Photophthalmia
(Arc Eye, Flash-Eye)

An industrial worker attends the ophthalmic emergency at midnight with acute pain in his eyes. There is a history of exposure to arc welding.

Ocular examination is simply not possible due to blepharospasm and edema of lids. Examination after topical anesthesia show conjunctival congestion with chemosis. Fluorescein stain is positive covering more than two-thirds of cornea.

Diagnosis: Industrial photophthalmia

INDUSTRIAL PHOTOPHTHALMIA

Industrial photophthalmia occurs by exposure of the eye to source of light rich in short waves used in many occupations such as flash light in cinematography, photograph, arc welding, tending in arc-furnaces and ultraviolet lamps and lights used in medical profession. The main factor responsible for photophthalmia is not wearing protective goggles and not using protective screens in the industries and occupations. Further, it is to be kept in mind that repeated small exposures over a period of 12 to 16 working hours are additive in effect. A cumulative 15 minutes exposure even at intervals would produce ocular symptoms of acute photophthalmia.

A study has shown that symptoms are produced by exposure to about 150 lumen/sq ft measured in terms of visible light. But a repeated exposure of cumulative 15 minutes from an arc light at a distance at which the intensity of light is only 10 lumen/sq ft will produce

photophthalmia. Thus, it is essential that the worker must protect himself with proper protective glass or screen. At the same time other persons must be advised not to look at the arc light even from a distance as repeated exposures from a distance also can cause photophthalmia.

Symptoms

There is a latent period of about 6 to 10 hours for the symptoms to manifest after exposure. Therefore, it is most usual for the symptoms to arise at midnight. The patient wakes up because of the symptoms. As symptoms are acute the patient has to attend the ophthalmic emergency at midnight.

The following symptoms are produced with varying intensity, depending upon the time and intensity of exposure to light.

With extreme intensity of exposure, the symptoms manifest in half an hour.

With less intensity the latent period may be long even 24 hours but never more than that as the factor of physiological repair counteracts the abiotic effect of the radiation.

If the intensity of radiation is weak and time of exposure is also short then such patient may just have a feeling of mild burning sensation with mild irritation.

- Sensation of a foreign body is the mildest symptom.
- Feeling of eyes full of sand particles is the moderate symptom.
- It follows with unbearable pain, lacrimation and marked blepharospasm.

- Followed by ciliary neuralgic pain.
- Patient is unable to bear even light from a night bulb or on effort to open the eyes.

Signs

- Lids are swollen.
- Conjunctiva is congested and chemosed.
- Fluorescein stain is positive.
- Pupil is miotic.

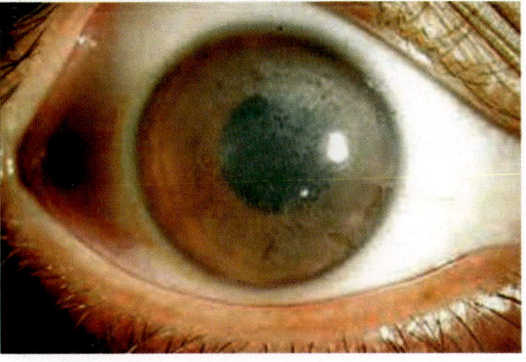

Fig. 39.1: Cornea epithelium denuded

Course

Normally the symptoms start subsiding after 48 hours with progress in the repair of the corneal epithelium which were destroyed due to abiotic effect of radiation. Even after complete healing and subsidence of symptoms, mild congestion and irritation persists for few days.

Management

- Provide relief from unbearable pain in the eyes and around.
- Instill topical anesthetic and examine the eye with the help of lid retractors.
- Stain to know the extent of damage to the corneal epithelium.
- Instill antibiotic eyedrops.
- Give bandage for 12 to 24 hours.
- Thereafter, instill topical antibiotic eyedrops six times a day for 10 days.

Assure the patient that he will get relief by the end of the day, i.e. after about 24 hours.

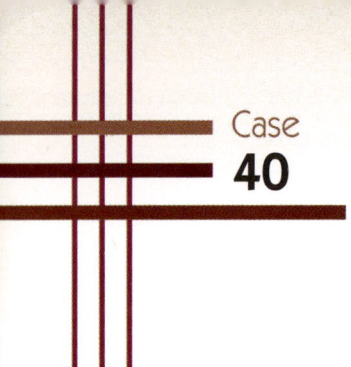

Plexiform Neurofibroma of Lid

A n adult male patient enters the clinic with thick, flabby and pendulous upper left lid hanging over the lower lid. Patient complains that his lid is full of long hard cords growing slowly for the last 3 years.

Ocular inspection shows a thick flabby pendulous left upper lid which is covering the eyeball and overhanging the lower lid. Patient is unable to lift the lid.

On palpation there is feeling of a bundle of hard cords locked in the bag.

Diagnosis: Plexiform neurofibroma of lid.

PLEXIFORM NEUROFIBROMA OF LID

The most characteristic manifestation of the plexiform neurofibroma is the palpebral form involving the upper lid (Fig. 40.1).

The lesion is present at birth and grows slowly and shows rapid growth with onset of puberty.

The most common site is within the distribution of the trigeminal and cervical nerves. The nerve most commonly involved is the supraorbital branches of the fifth nerve. Neurofibromata represents developmental defect of the neuroectodermal tissues with dominant inheritance.

Clinical Features

When the tumor is of considerable size then the involved lid appears thick, flabby, pendulous and overhanging the eyeball and the lower lid. Patient is unable to lift the lid. Examination of the eye cannot be conducted without use of lid retractors.

The overlying skin is normal and moves freely over the growth. Some cases may show thick, hyperelastic and coarse skin. The mass of the lid is soft to feel and is deeply fixed. On palpation the whole mass gives a feeling of a bag full of twisted hard and thick cords. The palpation is not tender. The swelling seems to be spreading over the frontotemporal region. It has a tendency to penetrate into the orbit causing proptosis.

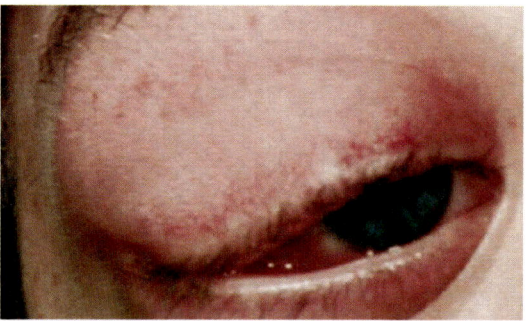

Fig. 40.1: Plexiform neurofibroma of lid

Management

The only treatment is surgical removal. It may be a problem if there is a deep penetration into the orbit. Patient may need a plastic reconstruction.

If the removal of mass is not complete then it can recur.

Part
3

Common Spot Diagnostic Cases

Congenital Cystic Eyeball

Grand mother with a baby in her lap enters the clinic with complaint of bulging of one eye in the child since birth. On examination, there is a bulge of the lower lid with a bluish cyst.

Diagnosis: Congenital cystic eyeball.

CONGENITAL CYSTIC EYEBALL

Congenital cystic eyeball is a condition which results due to a complete failure in the involution of the primary optic vesicle. The primary optic vesicle forms but fails to involute (so that the anterior part of the vesicle should come to lie in apposition with the posterior part of the vesicle, leaving merely a potential cleft between the two layers) and persists as a cyst replacing the eyeball. Sometimes the cyst is small and in that case the child presents clinically as a case of an anophthalmos. Usually, the cyst is large, even larger than a normal eyeball. This large cyst is a thin walled optic vesicle, appearing bluish in colour and occupies the centre of the orbit or shows bulge involving the upper lid or shows bulge involving the lower lid (Fig. 41.1).

Cyst may be single, or may be comprised of two or more loculi. The outer wall is of

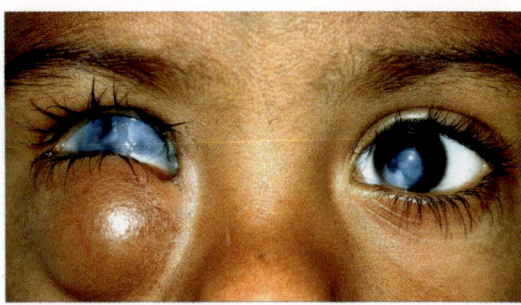

Fig 41.1: Congenital cystic eyeball—bulging lower lid

fibrous tissue representing the sclera. It is lined internally by the ectodermal tissue of the primary vesicle. Extraocular muscles may be inserted into the outer fibrous wall of the cyst. The cyst contains albuminous yellowish fluid. It is self-contained with no connection with the ventricular system of the brain.

Its etiology is unknown. There is no hereditary tendency. Most likely the environmental factor plays some role.

Treatment is surgical removal of the cyst. It should be followed by an acrylic prosthesis in the orbit. This will help the orbit to grow up to its normal size giving the child a good cosmetic appearance.

Anophthalmos/Microphthalmos

A n adult mother with baby in her lap enters the clinic with complaint of complete absence of one eye in her baby since birth.

On examination, the lid of one eye is caved in. On retraction of the lids, there is absence of eye.

Diagnosis: *Anophthalmos*.

ANOPHTHALMOS

Anophthalmos is a condition in which there is complete failure in the outgrowth of the primary optic vesicle, therefore, there is complete absence of tissues of the eye.

MICROPHTHALMOS

Microphthalmos is a condition in which the essential structure of the tissues of the eye are present, no matter how small the eye may be.

Clinically, it is quite impossible to differentiate anophthalmos from extreme microphthalmos. To make the matter simpler, a term 'clinical anophthalmos' has been used to designate majority of cases wherein the eye appears to be absent (Fig. 42.1).

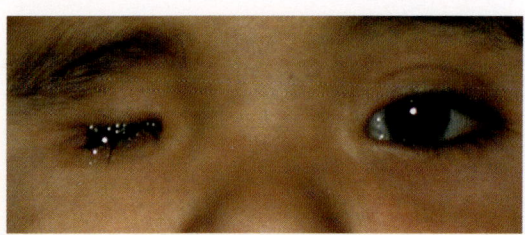

Fig. 42.1: Anophthalmos

Clinical Features and Management

- The external appearance of the child is normal.
- The orbit is well-formed but small.
- The palpebral and orbital tissues show disturbance in their balance of growth due to absence of the eye, though these are not dependent upon the optic vesicle for their differentiation.
- Lids are well-formed or to some extent rudimentary. In a case of anophthalmos, the lids are closed and caved in due to absence of eyeball. Examination is not possible without retraction of the lids.
- It may be associated with ankyloblepharon or epicanthus.
- Lids may show normal lashes, tarsal glands and lacrimal punctum. In some cases either the lashes or punctum may be absent.
- Shallow orbital cavity is lined by conjunctiva.
- Normal functioning lacrimal gland, confirmed by flow of tears when the child weeps.
- Extraocular muscles are present occasionally with normal innervation and power of contraction, but they are rarely sharply differentiated. These muscles either get inserted into subconjunctival tissue or into the rudimentary nodule.
- Optic canal is narrow or absent.
- Optic nerve is absent.
- Lower optic pathways and primary centres may be rudimentary or even aplasic or may be well-developed.

- If the child survives, then either the intellectual capacity is subnormal or may show complete idiocy.
- Association of anomalies have been reported in the form of a syndrome 'complicated anophthalmos of Francois' showing the anophthalmos with craniofacial deformity, hare-lip, polydactyly, cardiac anomalies and mental retardation.

Heredity

Most cases of anophthalmos occur sporadically.

It may show familial incidence occasionally.

Recessive genetic influence has been observed.

Sex-linked inheritance has been observed.

Consanguinity may play a part.

Hereditary factor is also suggested.

Sporadic occurrence of majority of cases of anophthalmos with no history of disease or consanguinity, is suggestive of environmental factor as a causative factor.

Involvement of the neural ectoderm is a prime factor.

Management

Aimed to provide cosmetic improvement.

An artificial eye cannot be provided due to small orbit and palpebral fissure.

The best plan is to enlarge the palpebral aperture by plastic surgery and at the same time put an acrylic prosthesis in the orbit.

If this procedure is undertaken at an early age, then the orbit can usually be enlarged to twice its original size in a short period.

Constant wear of a prosthesis is a must to maintain the growth of the orbit with growth of the child to provide him a good cosmetic appearance.

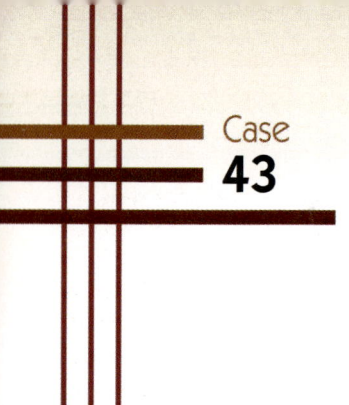

Epicanthus

arents attend the clinic with the complaint of internal squint in the child since birth.

On examination, there is a semilunar fold of skin running downwards at the side of nose with its concavity towards the inner canthus. The ocular movements are normal. The Hirschberg's test is normal. It is a case of an apparent internal squint.

Diagnosis: Simple epicanthus

EPICANTHUS

Epicanthus is a condition in which a semilunar fold of skin runs downwards at the side of the nose with its concavity towards the inner canthus (Fig. 43.1). It is a normal feature in fetal life from third to sixth month, in all the races. It tends to disappear in all the races, before birth, except in Mongols. Thus in the Mongols, the epicanthus remains permanently as a characteristic feature of that race. Presence of epicanthus is not uncommon in infancy, particularly when the nose is flat. It tends to disappear with the full development of the bridge of the nose at puberty. It tends to disappear rapidly in females than in males. It tends to persist to some extent in about 2 to 5% of cases.

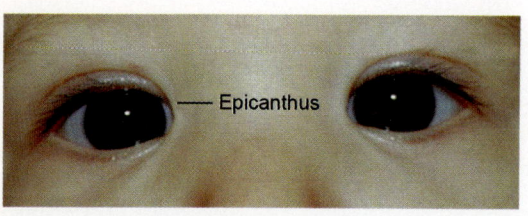

Fig. 43.1: Epicanthus

Epicanthus is invariably bilateral. The fold of the skin arises in the upper lid, runs down with crescentic course round the inner canthus and merges in the lower lid. The height and the width of the cresentic fold varies. A case with a broad epicanthal fold gives a characteristic appearance of Mongolian race with flat face, separated eyes, broad flat nose and an apparent internal squint. The appearance of the patient can be immediately improved just by pinching up the skin over the bridge of the nose into a fold. By this simple act, an eye physician can assure the parents that the appearance of the child shall become normal with the development of the bridge of the nose with age. It is gratifying.

Epicanthus with Ptosis

The association of ptosis with epicanthus is fairly common. In this condition, the males are affected twice as frequently as females. It is also commonly affected with disturbances of ocular motility, the common affection is internal strabismus and deficiency of upward movement. There is a strong hereditary tendency.

Epicanthus Inversus

Epicanthus inversus is associated with ptosis. This differs from the usual epicanthus. In this the skin fold arises in the lower lid and runs up crescentically upwards and merges itself in the upper lid. This fold does not override the inner canthus as in a usual type of epicanthus, but pushes the inner canthus outwards away for the nose, thereby causes shortening and deforming of the

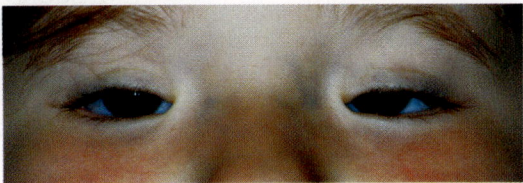

Fig. 43.2: Congenital ptosis with epicanthus inversus

palpebral aperture. There is a complete congenital ptosis due to aplasia of levator muscle.

ETIOLOGY

Simple epicanthus is transmitted as an autosomal dominant characteristic. Many cases show no hereditary tendency. No sex incidence.

TREATMENT

A case of simple epicanthus does not require any treatment. Just assure the parents that the child does not have any strabismus. The appearance of strabismus is false. The fold will disappear with the age with the full development of the bridge of the nose. Parents can be further assured by showing them, the effect of development of nose, just by pinching up the skin over the bridge of the nose into a fold. It will make the canthal fold disappear.

However, if the malady persists to some extent and the patient needs cosmetic improvement, then it can be corrected by surgery. A simple excision of a vertically elliptical area of skin in the region of the bridge of nose shall correct the malady. With modern methods of microsurgery, there is no reason to worry for a scar at the site of operation.

Epibulbar Dermoid

Patient presents with a small nodule at the limbus since birth.

On examination, there is a pinkish-yellow nodule with dry surface and few hairs.

Diagnosis: Epibulbar dermoid

Clinical Features and Management

- Common site for epibulbar dermoid is the limbus in the lower and outer quadrant (Fig. 44.1).
- Usually, it is unilateral. If bilateral then it will be placed symmetrically in both the eyes.

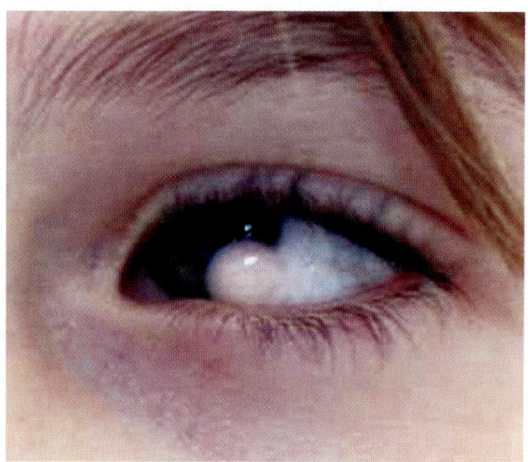

Fig. 44.1: Epibulbar dermoid

- Usually, it appears as round or oval nodule and may be pinkish-yellow in colour.
- Covered with dry conjunctiva and shows few short hairs on its surface.
- Usually, the dermoid is small in size. It may grow slowly and show fast growth at puberty.
- Fixed to the underlying tissue as the deeper layers are continuous with the corneal and scleral tissue.

Dermolipoma

Dermolipoma contains large amount of fatty tissue. These are small yellow tumors of congenital origin, frequently found subconjunctivally. The conjunctiva moves freely over these. Manifest anywhere, near limbus, at the inner angle, or between superior and lateral rectus muscles. These may be multiple. Most of these are of dermoid nature.

Management

Only treatment is the surgical removal of the dermoid. It is better to remove it at an early age and stage before it starts growing at puberty to provide good cosmetic appearance.

Removal in late stage leaves thick scar with cosmetic embarrassment.

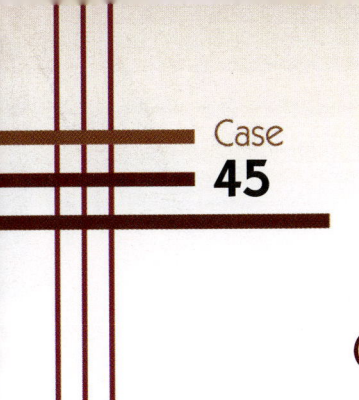

Orbital Emphysema

Young female professional enters the clinic with complain of slight bulging of the eye with swelling of the upper lid following a bout of sneezing in the morning. There is no pain or any other symptom.

Ocular examination shows slight proptosis of her left eye with marked swelling of the upper left lid. The lid appears puffy and soft. On palpation there are characteristic and diagnostic sign of crepitation.

Diagnosis: Orbital emphysema

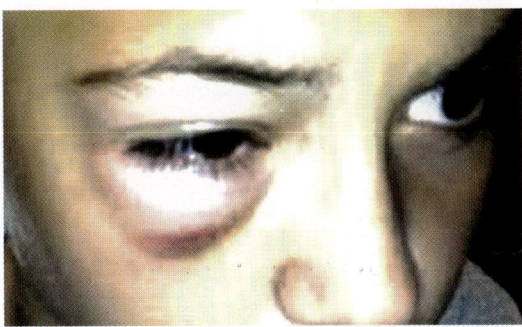

Fig. 45.1: Orbital emphysema

ORBITAL EMPHYSEMA

Emphysema is a condition wherein the air accumulates in the tissues of the lids and/or orbit.

Emphysema of lids and orbit indicates a communication with ethmoid sinus due to fracture of bony wall and rupture of mucosa.

Air accumulates typically on blowing the nose or on forceful sneezing.

Orbital emphysema is a rare condition but it has been observed in trivial trauma, postoperative trauma or even spontaneously. Even forceful sneeze or bout of sneezing is enough to produce orbital emphysema (Fig. 45.1).

Clinical Features and Management

Orbital emphysema occurs most commonly due to fracture of floor or inner wall of the orbit thereby communication is established between ethmoidal sinus and orbit.

Air collects in the orbital fatty tissue and muscle cone. The air from the orbit may traverse the tarso-orbital fascia and results in the emphysema of the lid.

Characteristic history from the patient leads to diagnosis.

Usual history is that the eye has bulged with swelling of the lid soon after a bout of forceful sneezing or blowing of the nose.

Proptosis and swelling of the lid reduces by pressure with characteristic feeling of crepitation (displacement of air).

One can, if careful, hear faint sound of crackling, or crunching like crunching of biscuit or potato chips.

Management

- Simple pressure bandage for a few hours is enough to displace the air. Total absorption of air takes a few days.
- *Percutaneous aspiration*: Decompression applied with 21 gauge needle under local anesthesia is effective and reliable technique in case with traumatic progressive orbital emphysema. Patient's discomfort decreases after the intervention.

Simple Coloboma of Iris
(Iridoschisma)

Most often a case of simple coloboma is encountered during routine clinical examination which shows a pear-shaped pupil in one or both the eyes.

Diagnosis: Simple coloboma of iris.

SIMPLE COLOBOMA OF IRIS

Clinical Features and Management

Simple coloboma of iris in the position of embryonic fissure (down and in) is termed as a 'typical coloboma of iris' and occurring elsewhere is termed as an 'atypical coloboma of iris' (Fig. 46.1). In fact, there is nothing fundamental in this distinction, as the iris is formed at a later date than the closure of the embryonic fissure.

Types of Coloboma

Total and Partial Coloboma

When the anomaly involves the whole sector of the iris up to the ciliary border then it is said to be 'total coloboma'.

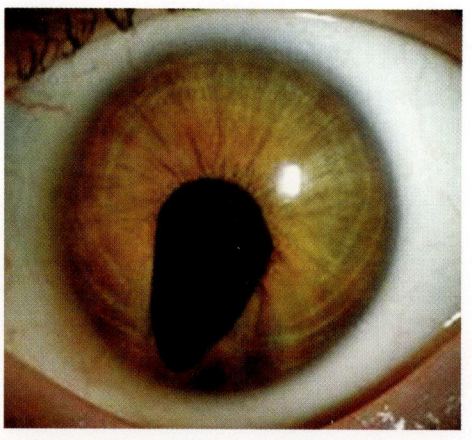

Fig. 46.1: Simple coloboma of iris

When the anomaly does not involve the whole sector of iris then it is said to be 'partial coloboma'.

Complete and Incomplete Coloboma (Pseudocoloboma)

When the anomaly involves the whole thickness of the iris then it is said to be 'complete coloboma'.

When the anomaly involves only the ectodermal or mesodermal layers of the iris then it is said to be 'incomplete coloboma' (pseudocoloboma).

Notch Coloboma

There is only a small notch in the pupillary margin.

Hole Coloboma

There is only a small hole in the substance of the iris.

Bridge Coloboma

There is a stretch of mesodermal tissue derived from the pupillary membrane across the coloboma.

Shape of Coloboma

Usually, it is pear-shaped with broad base towards the pupillary margin. It may be triangular or merely a narrow chink. It may have parallel sides or the sides may diverge peripherally.

Situation of Coloboma

It may be situated in any part of iris. Usually, it occurs with almost equal frequency downwards and inwards, downwards or downwards and outwards.

Heredity

The deformity is transmitted as an autosomal dominant characteristic.

Etiology

- *Most accepted Hess theory*: Growth of the iris is prevented by abnormally developed and persistent vascularized strands belonging to the fibrovascular sheath of the lens.
- Other view is that the coloboma may be considered as primarily an ectodermal defect of growth.

Features

- Simple coloboma of iris is one of the most common congenital abnormality of the eye appearing in about one in six thousand persons.
- Affects both the sexes equally.
- May be unilateral or bilateral.
- Does not affect the visual acuity.
- No cosmetic embarrassment.

Differential Daignosis from Surgical Coloboma

Clinically look and examine the collarette of the iris by slit lamp.

- In simple coloboma, the collarette can be traced up to the extreme periphery of the lower part of the coloboma along the pupillary border.
- In surgical coloboma, the collarette stops short at the cut edge of the iris.

Management

No cosmetic embarrassment so no management.

Oxycephaly (Acrocephaly, Tower Skull, Turricephally)

An adult male presents with proptosis, dim vision with vertically elongated skull an appearance which certainly attracts the attention.

On examination, the visual acuity in both the eyes is 6/18. There is pseudo-proptosis.

Ophthalmoscopy shows pale disk.

The vertex is dome-shape with a flat forehead and absence of superciliary arches.

Diagnosis: Oxycephaly

OXYCEPHALY

Oxycephaly is an anomaly which is characterized by a vertically elongated head with short transverse and anteroposterior measurements of the skull.

Oxycephaly is developmental anomaly due to defect in the primitive mesoderm which determines the bony structure of the skull (Fig. 47.1).

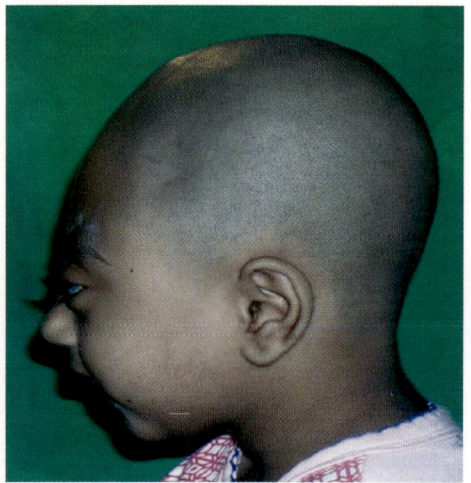

Fig. 47.1: Oxycephaly—tower skull

The deformity though evident at birth, develops during the first four years of life due to premature synostoses of skull sutures, restricting the growth of the base of the skull. The only space available for expansion of the brain is upwards thereby it assumes the shape of a tower skull that is vertically elongated head.

Clinical Features in a Typical Case

Features

- Vertically elongated skull.
- Flat vertical forehead.
- Absence of superciliary arches.
- Prominent nose.
- Small upper jaw.
- Heavy lower jaw.
- Narrow palate due to hypoplasia of maxilla.
- Orbits are shallow due to medial and forward displacement of the great wings of sphenoid.
- Roof of the orbit is almost vertical.
- Pituitary fossa is extremely narrow.
- Patient is likely to be mentally inefficient.

Ocular Symptoms

The ocular symptoms are secondary to bony deformity therefore symptoms tend to be progressive at first and later become stabilized with cessation of the growth of the brain.

- *Proptosis*: It is present in more than 50% of cases as a prominent ocular symptom. It is due to shallowness of the orbit.
- *Strabismus*: It is invariably divergent strabismus. It is due to low vision.

- *Nystagmus*: Patient may present with nystagmus.
- *Ocular movements*: Restriction of ocular movements again due to shallowness of the orbit.
- *Visual failure*: There may be loss of vision due to papilledema followed by optic atrophy. It is due to narrow optic canal, increased intracranial pressure and upward deflection of the optic nerve. The loss of vision occurs early and is seen in most of the cases. Fortunately the total loss of vision is rare.
- *Headache*: It may be due to raised intracranial pressure.

Management

Most of the cases live a useful life with workable vision. If there are signs and symptoms of raised intracranial pressure with papilledema then surgical interference may be considered.

Jaw Winking Ptosis
(Marcus Gunn's Phenomenon)

Young mother enters the clinic with her newborn son three months of age. She has noticed peculiar movement of her son's left upper lid while breastfeeding. The left upper lid shows movements with sucking. She demonstrates this to the female eye physician.

Diagnosis: Jaw winking phenomenon

JAW WINKING PHENOMENON

Jaw winking phenomenon is the most common congenital synkinetic movement of the lid. This phenomenon is most marked and noticed by the mother when the child is in his infancy. She notices this rapid movement of the upper lid usually of one eye during breastfeeding. Most cases are brought to the eye physician at this early stage. Many cases never attend an ophthalmic clinic until adult age.

Clinical Features and Management

Features

Partial ptosis of one eye wherein the upper lid covers upper half of the cornea. On opening the jaw the drooping lid shoots upwards to a level higher than the opposite normal lid. This phenomenon of lid shooting upwards on opening the mouth (jaw) is utilized by the patient to look upwards. During looking upwards he opens his mouth to have a better vision. This shooting upwards of the lid is not maintained if the mouth is kept open (Fig. 8.1).

There are various combinations and conditions in which the lid shows upward movement.

- Jaw movement in opposite side.
- Grinding movement of jaw.
- Forward protrusion of the jaw.
- On opening and closing the mouth.
- Not on opening the jaw but when the jaw is closed.
- On protrusion of tongue.
- On inspiration and opening the jaw.

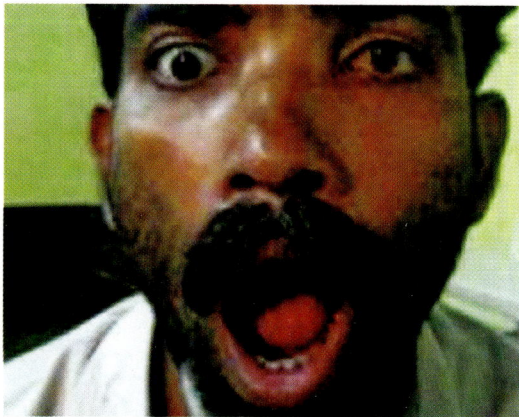

Fig. 48.1: On opening jaw—the partial ptosis right lid shoots up more than normal left lid

Etiology

There is abnormal nervous connection in the central nervous system between the nerve supply of the levator and the associated muscle. Thus, in the jaw winking phenomenon the levator has connection with third nerve nucleus and also with external pterygoid portion of the fifth nucleus.

Management

- Case with minor degree of anomaly does not require any treatment.
- Treatment, if desired, is surgical. The most effective surgical treatment is complete section of the levator thereby its action is abolished. Thereafter, treat the case as a case of ptosis, utilizing superior rectus muscle to raise and control the lid.

Albinotic Eye

Student of 10th standard complaints of low vision, dazzling, photophobia and constant movement of his eyes. Ocular examination shows white eyebrows and eyelashes. There is nystagmus. The pupil is red.

Diagnosis: An albinotic eye.

ALBINOTIC EYE

Albinism is a condition of a congenital deficiency of pigment. This is due to an 'inborn error of metabolism' characterized by the lack of the enzyme, tyrosinase, which converts 'DOPA' into melanin. Partial types of albinism are probably due to some functional insufficiency or defect in the distribution.

Clinical Features and Management

Features

The following features are seen in a case with albinotic eye:

- The eyebrows and eyelashes are white.
- Iris may appear pink because of increased transmission of light (Fig. 49.1).

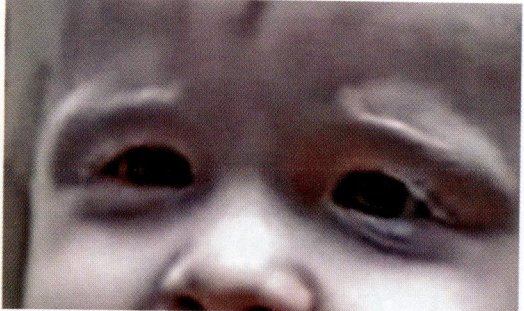

Fig. 49.1: Albino

- The pupil is red, as the light passing through the iris and sclera is reflected back from the choroidal vessels.

Ophthalmoscopy

- The fundus appears orange-red in colour (Fig. 49.2).
- Retinal and choroidal vessels are seen against the white sclera.
- Optic disk is visible as a point of confluence of retinal vessels.
- Macula is absent.

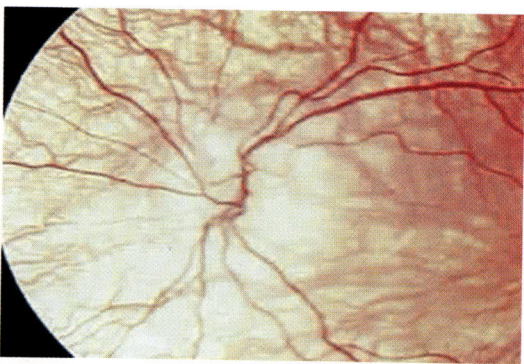

Fig. 49.2: Albinotic fundus

Other Features

- *Low vision*: It is due to presence of myopia and absence of macula or mal-development of macula.
- *Nystagmus*: It is a constant feature due to defective macula. Patient may have associated oscillatory head movements.

- *Photophobia*: It is due to excess of diffuse light entering the eye through the sclera.

Management

The only treatment to provide relief from photophobia and dazzling is wearing dark glass or sun goggles, with or without side-pieces to cut-out the lateral light entering the eye. Tinted soft contact lens can be used. Correct the refractive error. Nystagmus can be treated surgically by weakening the muscles responsible for the slow movement. A bilateral recession, may be reasonably helpful.

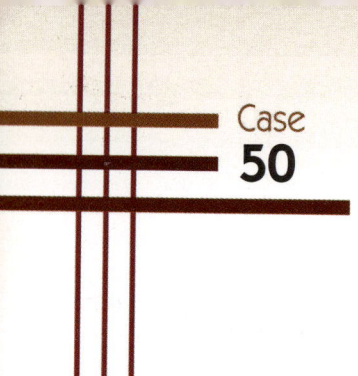

Buphthalmos

A mother enters the clinic with her child about one year-old in her lap. She points towards the enlarged left eyeball which is protruding forward. The child is unable to open the eye and is definitely seeing much less. Ocular examination shows an enlarged globe with large globular cornea which is hazy.

Diagnosis: Buphthalmos

BUPHTHALMOS

Buphthalmos is a condition of congenital glaucoma due to obstruction of drainage of intraocular fluid through the angle. It is a developmental anomaly.

CLINICAL FEATURES AND MANAGEMENT

Features

The most characteristic features of the buphthalmic eye (Fig. 50.1) are as follows:

- Whole globe is enlarged giving it a clinical picture of proptosis.
- Cornea is globular in shape, with diameter of more than 12 mm.

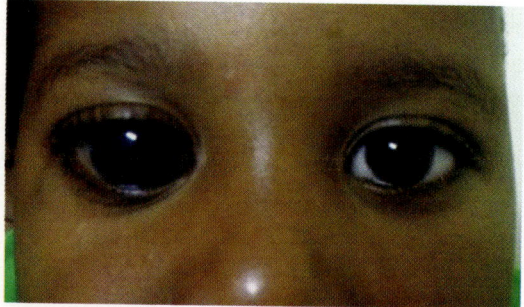

Fig. 50.1: Right eye buphthalmos

- Sclera appears blue due to stretching.
- Anterior chamber is deep.
- Iris may be tremulous due to lack of support from the lens.
- Lens is pulled backwards due to stretching of the zonules.
- Lens may be subluxated.
- Cornea appears hazy due to rupture of Descemet's membrane.
- Cornea appears hazy due to epithelial edema if the intraocular pressure is raised.
- Cornea may ultimately become porcelain-white in appearance and its sensation is lost.
- Ophthalmoscopy if possible may show a cupping of the disk.
- Angle of the anterior chamber shows developmental anomalies.

Symptoms

There is a triad of symptoms in a typical case:

1. Photophobia.
2. Blepharospasm.
3. Epiphora.

Any infant, if presents with the above symptoms then carefully exclude buphthalmos because these symptoms appear before the characteristic signs of enlargement of the globe and large and hazy cornea manifest.

With the manifestation of buphthalmos above symptoms become much more in intensity.

The photophobia is distressing and due to this the infant likes to keep the face burried in the 'pallu' (part of saree which hangs downwards) of his mother.

Differential Diagnosis

- Anterior megalophthalmos.
- High congenital myopia.
- Congenital staphylomata.
- Congenital hereditary dystrophies.
- Corneal edema may occur following trauma, raised pressure and inflammation of cornea.

Management

Treatment is primarily surgical. The best results have been obtained by:

- Goniotomy
- Goniotomy combined with goniopuncture.
- Until the patient is taken for surgery, medical therapy should be given to control the intraocular pressure.
- Surgical treatment should not be delayed once the diagnosis is confirmed.
- An early surgery saves the eye and the vision.

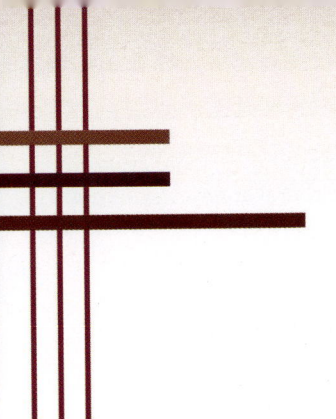

Index